Understanding Advanced Hypnotic Language Patterns

A Comprehensive Guide

John Burton, EdD

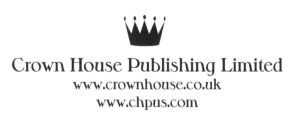

Crown House Publishing Limited

www.crownhouse.co.uk
www.chpus.com

First published by

Crown House Publishing Ltd
Crown Buildings, Bancyfelin, Carmarthen, Wales, SA33 5ND, UK
www.crownhouse.co.uk

and

Crown House Publishing Ltd
6 Trowbridge Drive, Suite 5, Bethel, CT 06801-2858, USA
www.chpus.com

British Library of Cataloguing-in-Publication Data
A catalogue entry for this book is available
from the British Library.

10-Digit ISBN: 1845900324

13-Digit ISBN 978-1845900328

LCCN 2006934876

Contents

Acknowledgments

There are many people I want to thank for contributing to this material and eventual book. I thank my clients for their courage to change themselves and their lives. I appreciate their trust in me to assist in this effort. I also want to thank Crown House Publishing and the staff for their willingness to publish my manuscript and the skillful editors who helped me present this material in a more effective manner. Thanks to Steve Lankton for his skill and generosity. Many thanks also to friends and colleagues who contributed their awareness, support, and encouragement.

Through this process of conducting therapy, promoting change in others, and the materials and tools utilized, there is a theme of trust. Yes, trust of client toward therapist, and in addition, trust of therapist in self, and then, trust of client in self. This overriding theme of trust grants access to and use of higher levels of self. Thus, I express appreciation for the powers of trust and what this grants as we gain the resources and resulting experiences we most deeply desire. Lastly and most deeply I express appreciation for the One who makes all things possible.

John Burton

Introduction
Hypnotic Language:
A Cognitive–Developmental
Approach

In this work, we will explore hypnotic language through several perspectives. The primary emphasis will come from a cognitive point of view. This cognitive view includes thinking styles and human development levels, as well as levels of perception. And just what is hypnotic language, you may ask. Hypnotic language involves structuring sentences in such a way as to invite the reader or listener into a trance state. Here we will define a trance state as being a heightened state of focus or concentration on a single item or group of like items to the exclusion of all other items.

The principal purpose of hypnotic language, according to this work, is to assist clients into a trance for the purposes of examining the contents of a particular focus, allowing the clients to then adjust the contents, meaning, and influence in their life. The development and study of hypnotic language stems primarily from the work of Milton Erickson, MD. My hope is that this present work will add to the understanding of the structure and therapeutic applications of hypnotic language.

Hypnotic language could be thought of as taking *three* general forms. The first form addresses the cognitive aspects of a person's experience. This includes rather directly accessing cognitive styles, including the developmental and perceptual ingredients that create one's experience. In essence, this form of hypnotic language attempts to restructure an individual's experience and the meaning attached to the experience. Addressing cognitive aspects of one's experience amounts to reframing by dismantling and reconstructing the ingredients making up the frame that sets the experience.

The second form of hypnotic language might be thought of as metaphorical forms of communicating with the unconscious mind.

This communication is offered to the client while they are in a more formal trance. The method of change here occurs through helping the client recategorize experiences. This also becomes reframing. But a different path to reframing is taken in this second form. While the cognitive approach addresses the parts that make up the frame, the metaphorical path works by addressing the frame as a whole, and then moving the contents into another frame to create new meaning.

By way of a metaphor to distinguish between these two hypnotic language forms: sometimes people remodel their house, giving it a whole new feel, whilst sometimes in order to give it a whole new feel, people move their entire house to a new location.

A third type of hypnotic language works by bringing a needed but missing resource to the situation, bringing the mountain to Mohammed, so to speak. This third style of hypnotic language assists personal change by introducing awareness of new resources into an existing frame. Once introduced and integrated, the new resource then creates a whole new frame and eventually a different emotional-behavioral outcome. The avenue for introducing this new resource is also a metaphorical one, presented while the client is in some degree of trance.

The first section of this book presents a model that describes how we cognitively process information. We'll use this model to explain the layers and stages of information processing. This four-tier hierarchy of information processing will also serve to identify the cognitive targets of hypnotic language.

Now we will move to describing the four-tier structure involved in cognitive processing of information. These four tiers will be discussed in more detail in subsequent chapters. But for now, here is a general thumbnail sketch of each tier and its role. The first tier of this four-tier system comes into play when we experience a stimulus. Initially, we receive information through one or more of our five senses. This information may come from observing or interacting with external sources. We may also receive information through internal sources such as bodily sensations. This information received from one or more of our senses sends signals to our brain and the information is subjected to the dynamics of the first tier of the hierarchy.

The first tier of the information-processing system is referred to here as the continuum of awareness. The continuum of awareness consists of levels of awareness based on the amount of comparative information we use when assessing a stimulus. This continuum determines the general frame size we notice. This general frame is made up of the available information to use when comparing, contrasting, and then processing the new stimulus into a meaningful subset of a whole.

The second tier of this meaning-making process involves putting the sorted information together into some organized meaning in relation to other parts, somewhat like assembling a jigsaw puzzle. Frames or categories of information are created here. I use the terms frames and categories as having the same meaning in this work. This information-assembling process involves Gestalt psychology categories of frame making or categorizing information. We assemble initially random pieces of information into some meaningful, relatively sensible whole by using the parts of the puzzle. It is interesting to note that the available parts of the puzzle stem from the level of awareness within the continuum of awareness, and the perceptual-cognitive level of development used when sorting the information. This meaning-making event is an interaction effect between the perceptual-cognitive level of development and Gestalt framing mechanisms.

The third tier consists of processes that attempt to make more personal meaning of the information received through our senses (Keagan, 1983). This process consists of sorting the received information through one of several perceptual and cognitive levels of development (Piaget, 1965). To a great extent, the perceptual-cognitive level through which the information is sorted determines its potential meaning in our lives. This potential meaning ranges from self-limiting beliefs to unlimited possibilities for success. Once the information received gets identified, a function of our perceptual-cognitive-developmental level, we send the labeled pieces to the next tier of the hierarchy for further meaningful assembly.

To give an example that may help solidify these first three levels of perceptual-cognitive development concepts, imagine walking into a clothing store. You decide to sort through the collection of clothing for red shirts. You filter out all other shirts as well as all other clothing. But you could then decide you want to sort for the whole range of reds from pink to maroon. Perhaps you then decide to sort for all light-colored shirts and then all shirts. And since you are in the clothing store anyway, you then decide to open up your perception to notice all clothing, then to what other clothing exists, not just in this store, but in other stores, and even what has yet to be designed and created. With this last level of awareness, you reach the apex of perceptual-cognitive development that contains all possibilities, known or otherwise.

One could easily make the argument that the second and third processing factors, perceptual and cognitive principles, exist at the same level of the hierarchy. But I would suggest that we first must sort sensory information depending on our perceptual level since the perceptual level determines what and how much we can notice. We then make use of this perceptually influenced material with our cognitive and meaning-making skills to weave it into some sort of meaningful frame. In another analogy, you might think of this whole multilevel process as resembling collecting numbers. The perceptual level determines which numbers we notice. The Gestalt framing process then adds up these numbers to find the sum total. The cognitive sorting process then sorts to determine the meaning of this sum total to self, others, and life. This last step comes into being as a consequence of available ingredients. It seems we feel compelled to organize and make meaning of our experiences in life. Even if the information is disparate, we force fit the information into some category.

In this model, the fourth and highest level of information processing really exists as a sort of two-headed being. Depending on how we approach and utilize this duo, it can be a two-headed monster or a two-headed omnipotent ruler. The two heads—for better or worse—that I refer to here are states of emotion and personal beliefs. States of emotion and personal beliefs exist in an inseparable form, somewhat like mind-body. They agree with or mirror each other, as these two forces naturally reflect one another.

States of emotion and beliefs have a significant effect on how we process information. These two variables, states and beliefs, operate as self-sustaining entities. Like politicians, once a state or belief is in place it does all it can to stay there. States and beliefs tend to function as self-fulfilling prophecies. We usually filter the information we find within the general frame, assemble it, and then add meaning in accordance with the state of our emotions and beliefs. This alliance between the four tiers creates a sort of meta-Gestalt all its own and can be very difficult to separate back into parts that can be interpreted and utilized independently.

This unique interpretation of the parts within the meta-gestalt can allow freedom through new awareness, gestalts, meanings, states, and beliefs. Interestingly, we do the same process in reverse to the existing information in the meta-gestalt to disassemble it as we did to assemble it. In other words, we no longer permit the meta-gestalt to exist separate from the larger whole. We create this return to the whole by drawing on an expanded continuum of awareness, "gestalting" cognitive processing, as well as beliefs and states of emotion. Once returned to the whole, a whole new meaning can evolve that more effectively serves one's highest purpose. Hypnotic language is one of the ways of undoing and re-creating the meaning-making process, ending up with more effective life choices.

Examining the influence of states and beliefs further, if a person experiences a state of sadness, he almost certainly also holds a correspondingly gloomy belief about self, life, or others. Conversely, if a person believes that she is competent, her state will reflect this belief, and she will exhibit confidence, or some state similar to confidence. If the two factors, emotions and beliefs, are at odds, this results in a form of cognitive dissonance (Festinger, 1957), treated as an internal conflict between emotional states, beliefs, and values.

Chapter 1
Categorizing Data:
The Continuum of Awareness

This chapter concerns how we categorize information in our lives and will serve as a more general template through which to view hypnotic language and cognitive processes. The continuum of awareness, as referenced here, represents the first of the four tiers within the information-processing system. Whether we receive information from the environment through our senses or we just experience from within, we naturally categorize the information we notice. When categorizing information, we seem to draw from a pre-existing category based on similarities between the new information and the existing category. We then place the "new" experience within the closest matching category.

Categorizing is all about comparing pieces of information and their details. We compare the information on which we focus to other known information in order to determine in which category the information belongs. This begs the question of what will we do with truly new or unique information that does not relate to other already known information. Here we may delete, distort, or generalize to force fit an item into an old category or seize the opportunity for a unique experience.

I suggest that fear limits anyone's openness to truly new experiences. By doing what Gestalt psychology calls simplifying, we think we better protect ourselves by deleting, distorting, and generalizing new experiences so that they resemble familiar ones. But excluding the uniqueness of experiences actually endangers us more instead of protecting us. By noticing uniqueness we find more possibilities and opportunities for solutions and effective self-directing. In other words, fear may lead us to a closed-minded style of thinking that limits awareness of choice, making our fears come true. Part of the challenge to overcoming this limiting fear is bypassing conscious efforts at categorizing.

In some sense, hypnotic language attempts to defy conscious mind categorizing, giving the information within the hypnotic language uniqueness, and thus promoting new awareness and new responses to life. Focusing further on language, there seems to be some interesting parallels between language and other concepts. First, language appears to be the result of a deductive process. We begin with a general concept or idea about something. We then find and use words that we hope describe this idea, just as I am doing here.

When attempting to communicate, I reduce my ideas to a sequence of words that attempt to convey these ideas as well as my abilities permit. Yet these words come from a larger pool of words, a dictionary of sorts. We use words to describe other words, involved in a rather circular process so long as we use words. When we just think, feel, and then experience, we can leave words behind and simply experience. But to describe what we experience, we resort to words, actually reducing the experience by categorizing through words. Essentially, words can become a vehicle transporting us to a place of unmediated experience, which can allow more creative, resourceful living.

At the same time that all words stem from a common, all-inclusive word pool, words also resemble numbers in some ways. Years ago, I used to think of the number zero as actually being the circle, O. Later I came to realize that the circle is not zero; the line is a circle. The zero is the content of the circle, the nothing. (Bear with me, as there is a method to this apparent madness.) All numbers, then, are essentially units away from this zero, this nothing. A positive 12 is 12 units away from zero. A negative 424 is this many units away from zero in the other direction. Just as words use other words to describe them, numbers use a common reference, zero. Words and numbers both come from a common pool.

Words use other words to describe a concept. We use a part of the whole of all words to describe another part of the whole of all words. We may also then use a part, words, to describe a larger concept, a metaphor, for example. We may also use words to refer to the entirety of all concepts, the one or the whole, in some philosophical sense. This highest level of awareness perhaps consists of all resources in their yet to be activated or utilized forms. These concepts or resources reside in the whole and resemble the entire raw number system that can be utilized as we most resourcefully desire. Let us not get bogged down in this philosophical discussion.

My point is that numbers and language have a common structure. Each derives from a common source, and this common source is both nothing and everything at the same time: It contains all possibilities and resources. By utilizing hypnotic language, a person can access this unstructured whole, which then permits creation of a more beneficial structure for living. Generally, hypnotic language represents just one of many vehicles through which one can increase awareness and reap the benefits this brings to life.

This introduction to words, numbers, and the concept of a sliding scale, from singular awareness to awareness of a whole, now leads us to what I refer to as the continuum of awareness. The process of change that can occur through hypnotic language will then be demonstrated within this awareness continuum. As previously stated, how we categorize data will serve as this book's larger framework or template through which to view an individual's thinking process and to assess their potential well-being. I suggest that these ways of categorizing data comprise general levels of perception and that the level of perception from which we experience life actually determines our experience of life.

The ideas presented here about perception are reminiscent of Victor Frankl's (1973) existentially based Logotherapy. It is my belief that what we experience in life results from our perceptual position along an ever-increasing awareness scale. Experience inside our self stems from what we are able to perceive, either within or outside the self. This perception then determines the proportion of the whole of which we are aware and largely dictates response options. We often make the mistake of believing the level of perception from which we live is the only one in existence. This leads to emotional, behavioral, and physical problems.

I also suggest that problems stem from and are a byproduct of our level of perception, not the result of an event that "happens" to us. We may say that we experience emotional hurt as the result of some event. I will offer a process definition of emotional hurt. I propose that emotional hurt is a process whereby one withholds from oneself a beneficial resource-state in response to an event. This state could be joy, assertiveness, determination, or some state that permits effective, satisfying living. It is the withholding of the resource that brings the sense of hurt rather than the actual event. For example, we experience emotional hurt in response to withholding of joy from the self. This accidental self-denial of a resource stems from the belief formed at a particular perceptual position (Burton, 2003). Therefore, emotional hurt results from one's perceptual position, occurring solely within the individual. Ultimately therapy—whether hypnotherapy or any effective therapy—aims to elevate the perceptual position of the client and allow recategorizing of information from a hurtful category to a benign or resourceful category.

Since categorizing information involves comparing at least two pieces of information, the size of the comparison chunk—quality—and the number of chunks—quantity—play a significant role in determining how we categorize data. The quality of a comparison determines its significance, whether it is minor or major and just how many instances of this experience exist in this category. The more emotionally charged the category and/or the more examples of the category, the more power it exerts in categorizing new information. The quantity of information chunks determines how many different pieces of information we use when comparing new to existing information. When we just look at similarities, we limit the effectiveness of our categorizing. In looking at differences and parts of the whole, we find their independent uniqueness and perhaps more effective uses in new experiences.

This categorizing process largely determines our emotional states and the noticed response options. I emphasize "noticed response options". All response options exist simultaneously; we just *notice* the ones corresponding to our level of awareness. You can equate level of awareness with the term perception, since our level of awareness determines what and how we perceive. In cognitive psychology, the premise is that our thoughts determine our emotions. I would modify this by stating that our perceptual position determines our thoughts. Therefore, our perceptual position determines our emotions.

Here is a simple example of perceptual position or perceptual level and its influence on our thoughts and emotions. If we see the color red and then just compare it to blue, we may say that red is not blue and blue is not red. But we leave out the roughly seven million colors that our eyes can perceive. If I want to paint my living room, I may only notice two options, blue and red. Maybe I'm frustrated because I feel restricted. Maybe later I notice the color yellow and expand my options, but remain unaware of the wide range resulting from these primary colors. When I finally become aware of the full spectrum of colors, and thus of potential choice, maybe I will likely feel a sense of freedom and excitement about this and the spectrum of choices I now recognize.

Any given perceptual level generally determines what we notice, available response options, and then, to some extent, the general range of consequences on our lives. I suggest that the therapeutic premise within counseling is that, by increasing awareness, we may then utilize a larger category of data when examining a specific element in life. Acknowledging this larger—hopefully largest—category of data as a comparison base naturally leads us to more available meanings, response options, and more beneficial life consequences.

Using the largest comparison base—all the colors of the spectrum, for example, to assess a specific element in life, living room color—may not seem especially significant. Still, this comparison of a single to the all-encompassing whole changes everything in its wake. It results in a potentially immediate shift in the meaning-making process, beliefs, and chosen states of emotion. In simple terms, you could call this expanding awareness gaining a better perspective.

I refer to the *range* of category size as the continuum of awareness. The continuum of awareness ranges from an all-or-nothing category to the infinite, all-inclusive whole. To represent the categories of the continuum, I borrowed the statistical categories of nominal, ordinal, interval, and ratio data. The essence of this continuum is that the larger the comparison group we use when assessing a single item of information, the greater our awareness, the more numerous our response options, and the greater our effectiveness in decision making.

Before going further, I'll cite a simple example using these four categories of data. We'll use a discussion between a teenager and his parents negotiating how late he can stay out with his friends. This boy, James, wants to stay out until midnight on Friday. His mother says no, he can stay out only until 10 o'clock. James says that his friend Richard gets to stay out until 1 a.m. This allows only one other comparison. His mother says that Richard may stay out until 1 a.m., but some children stay out until 9 p.m., while others stay out all night, and still others are not allowed to go out with their friends at all on Friday nights. This expanded awareness modifies the mentality-emotionality of James, leading to resolution.

We started with either/or, midnight, or 10 p.m., and then considered more and more possibilities until a whole range of possibilities came into awareness. This process of expanding awareness from either/or to the whole range of possibilities represents the process, influence, and benefits of using the continuum of awareness. Each successively larger category of awareness modifies our thinking, feeling, and decision making for the better.

The Four Categories of Awareness

1. **Nominal information** exists here in terms of all or nothing, the presence or absence of a trait—pregnant or not, for example. Nominal data equate to nominalizing information. This is a labeling process. Look for what and how a person labels self, others, events, or life. What group do they use for comparison purposes?

   Symptoms experienced as a result of relying on nominal data include anxiety and depression, as well as anger and hopelessness. A host of physical problems, including high blood pressure, headaches, and irritable bowel syndrome, may also result from living life from the level of nominal data level of awareness only. You may think this notion of physical symptoms resulting from how we categorize data a bit of a stretch. But how we categorize data largely determines our view of the world, then the choices we think we can make, and thus influences our physical state.

Think about someone who you know who experiences physical symptoms such as headaches, high blood pressure, or irritable bowel syndrome. Notice this individual's thinking style and how they categorize data. The mentality resulting from all-or-nothing thinking, reliance on nominal data, constricts a person mentally *and* physically, I believe. The physical conditions identified above may stem from some sort of physical constricting process, mirroring mental constriction. It often appears true that people who utilize nominal data find themselves in an ego-defensive position as they take events personally, egocentricity running their life's show.

As an example of nominal data in daily living, consider a woman who is interviewing for a job as an entry-level marketer for a large company. She is offered the job and can either accept it or turn it down. There are no other options at the moment within this frame. We will follow this woman and her roles within this company as an ongoing example of categories of data.

2. **Ordinal information**. Such data receive a simple rank order without reference to the distance between items. There is no zero in this category of data. A frame is set by ordinal data and information must come from within this frame. Ordinal data are displayed when ranking the order of participants in a race. This one is better than that one, but no reference is made to how much better; it is quantity without quality. Ranking the finishing order of the horses in a race is yet another example of ordinal data. There is a first and second place, along with third; the remaining participants are ranked as to their order of finish—hence ordinal data. Receiving letter grades for school courses also represents original data. If you come up with two response options to a situation, each supposedly within the framework of a particular desired outcome, you have framed the situation with ordinal data. In psychotherapy, double binds exemplify ordinal data. Speaking to a child about getting himself cleaned up, you ask, "Would you rather take a bath or a shower?"

Now I'll provide an example of ordinal data in action, using the woman who accepted the job as entry-level marketer. Let's first point out that ordinal data are quite restrictive. The ideas or options for a given situation must reside within the ordinal frame category. Our example: This woman now works at a large company as a marketer. She started at the entry level and moved up to junior level marketer, then to a senior marketing position. She is now being offered the position of Director of Marketing. The framework of this ordinal data is the category of marketing positions within the company. She can keep her current job role or accept a potentially better job as marketing director. But each job is within the frame and no zero—a job outside the marketing department—exists as an option. We'll follow-up on this example in the next category of data to see how interval data expand possibilities.

Ordinal data leave many blanks between each item in a given list and ranking. In some ways, ordinal data simply organize nominal data, leaving out fluidity and flexibility. Ordinal data restrict the range of response options to just a single category. This single category of data can also play out in self-limiting ways. If we have already decided that we will fail at an opportunity, all resources become subjected to the overall category called "ways to fail". In other words, ordinal data may represent a belief about self, life, or others; we then select the option that self-fulfills this prophecy.

In some ways you might think of ordinal data as representing small picture thinking. The category is selected first and then the application is made rather than assessing the big picture and then choosing the appropriate category. With ordinal data we decide the category and how we will measure the elements within it and then work within these parameters. This concept sounds restrictive, doesn't it? It can be if it does not first result from examining the whole or the big picture. In other words, if you begin a project by deciding you must incorporate some particular element, then you are using nominal data; the tail is wagging the dog. If you decide that you know of some variation of this particular element that is better than the initial one, yet still an example of the item, that is ordinal thinking.

Change comes to ordinal data and ordinal thinking by shifting and generalizing one's focus. If you first decide what outcome you want, then any and all similar functioning elements become known and available for use. For example, I want to hang a painting on my wall. I have the picture hanger with the nail ready to go. But I do not have a tool to drive the nail into the wall. If I believe I must use a hammer, then I restrict myself to ordinal data. I believe I must find a hammer of some sort to use. But thinking outside the ordinal box I can then find any item that is solid and heavy enough to serve the purpose of driving the nail into the wall. If I get even further outside the ordinal box, I find that any solid object with a flat surface bigger than the nail head can be used to simply push the nail through the *sheetrock*. I have used many items over the years, including the flat edge of a car key, to push nails into *sheetrock*. By focusing on the general function desired, numerous items become available that effectively perform the function.

3. **Interval information**. In this category, the trait is present in each item, is ranked, and the distance or degree of the trait between each item is noted—hence interval data. A zero exists here but has no meaning beyond the absence of the trait. Weight and time are examples of interval data. You can possess more time but there is only so much time you can have.

Weightless is the least we can weigh. Test scores, 0–100, and humidity, 0–100, are also examples of interval data. Language using interval data does not manifest itself in the true form of a double bind. It may resemble what could be called a triple bind, with the zero, an absence of trait-behavior, taking the form of an undesirable outcome. Speaking to the child about cleaning himself up, you say: "Would you rather take a bath of shower, or just stay dirty, and have the other kids wonder why you smell funny?"

Let's return to the example of the woman working as a marketer. With ordinal data she was faced with choosing a job within the marketing department. Now, with interval data, jobs outside the marketing department come into awareness as a zero—no marketing role exists. Maybe these jobs outside the marketing department exist in this same company, perhaps within the human resource department, the advertising department, or some other section of the company. She can rank order the marketing jobs, senior versus director, and then include other job opportunities outside of marketing. Yes, the larger frame of jobs within the company still rules but the options expand to jobs outside the marketing department.

In displays of self-limiting interval data, you may still hold the belief that you will fail at some task but now, with interval data, there exist an increased number of ways of failing, such as doing nothing at all toward a task, rather than actively behaving in ways that bring about failure.

It is also interesting to note that temperature is not on the interval data scale. While absolute zero exists, –459° Fahrenheit (–273° Celsius), the other extreme, heat, is not really known, perhaps not even measurable. With temperature there is a range and zero has meaning; it is not the absence of the quality measured, which is temperature in this case. By now you may be asking yourself, why are we being given this information?

I present this information about temperature and other ways of measuring to begin expanding awareness not only of this category's limits but also to begin pondering what resides beyond these limits, thus leading to open-ended ratio data.

4. **Ratio information**. Here we confront the most complex data. Here an identified trait is present and ranked, with a relationship between items noted. This category adds the dimension of a true zero that has meaning. Examples include the number system, plus and minus infinity. The place of pure potentiality, the totality of everything in the universe makes up this category of data.

Let's look at the woman in the marketing position within the large company from a ratio data perspective. She first took the job offer rather than turn it down as an example of nominal data. She was then offered a job promotion from a senior marketing position to that of Director of Marketing, as an example of ordinal data. She subsequently realized other employment possibilities existed within the company, such as human resources or advertising, representing interval data. Now, thinking more deeply, she becomes aware that her true desire is to own and run a bakery and catering business. She has stepped out of interval data and into ratio data by considering data possibilities outside the narrow confines of the first three data frames. She opens herself up to broader, more free-ranging alternatives that permit more satisfying choices and solutions by entering the ratio level of awareness.

There are several significant influences arising from these four categories of data and how we use them. These ever-expanding categories, from nominal through ratio data, form a sort of funnel shape, representing our degree of awareness (see Figure 1:1). At the lower end of the funnel, the narrowest portion, we find our most narrow awareness, nominal data, followed by ordinal, interval, and ratio, in ascending order.

Figure 1:1   *The Continuum of Awareness*

As stated earlier, it seems that the general purpose of counseling or psychotherapy is to help move a person's awareness from a narrower to a broader perspective. The purpose of such movement is to help the client become aware of different perceptions, beliefs, resource states, and options. With such awareness they will be enabled to make constructive and effective choices to achieve personal goals. The general goal for making use of this continuum is learning how to live at the top and just visit the bottom while taking action. The lowest level exists just as the point of implementation of personal action plans. Many people live at the lower level and only occasionally visit the upper level. Ideally, we reverse this, living at the upper level and only visiting the lower. The lower level is fraught with confusing illusions due to constricted perception. When we visit the lower level, we need to carry with us a clear blueprint of overall awareness, so that we do not come to believe in and be entrapped at the lower level.

Going Up?

Our response to circumstances stems from the perceptual level on which we operate. The lower levels are noisier, asking for more attention to countless distracting details. As a result, we often feel drawn down to them and act from there, but this is restrictive and often not effective. It often seems our first response to distress is to dive to a lower level of perception, believing there we get a closer look and maybe construct a better defense. Unfortunately, this lower level increases our distress and decreases our effectiveness in responding. The more effective response will likely mean rising above the level of the distress, finding a broader awareness, and a more effective, less distressed response. The moral here is to do the opposite of what is first noticed: go up the perceptual ladder, not down, leaving the emotionally noisy lower basement and ascending to the tower and observe more and better, choosing a more effective response and utilizing foresight, patience, and flexibility.

I'll use a brief example of hypnotic language to illustrate the levels of data and how they manifest in words. This example displays the dynamics of each level and is intended to give you a feel for the influence of gradually expanding your awareness. I used this relaxation language pattern with a client who described his thoughts as racing. I asked him which one (of his thoughts) was winning, to inject some humor and loosen his state of anxiety. I then went on to use the car and driving theme as an entry into the language pattern below. I indicate where the particular continuum-data categories begin by using parentheses.

> (**Nominal level**) Have you ever been riding in a car—who knows where you were exactly, but you were a passenger in the car, maybe in the front seat—and you were just looking out the window down at the roadside, watching the edge of the road as you passed along? You noticed how incredibly fast the road passed beneath you, how landmark after landmark flew by. It seemed extremely fast. (**Ordinal level**) Then maybe you decided to look just a bit further off the road, maybe to a front yard as you passed by. And then the next front yard as you passed, noticing that the yards passed by more slowly, it took longer for them to go by or really for you to go by them. (**Interval level**) And then maybe you decided to look even further off the roadside and notice the houses, or beyond these, behind the houses.

And you noticed how much more slowly these passed, or you actually passed them. This seems much slower and (**Ratio level**) then you decided to look even further off in the distance, perhaps to the uttermost edge of the horizon or maybe up at a cloud in the sky, way off in the distance. You know how clouds can sometimes appear in the shape of something else familiar, like a dog or a boat or something else? And you can stare at a cloud way off in the distance, not really knowing quite what shape it is taking but also noticing that it seems to be completely still, not moving at all, and how paradoxical this stillness feels. You know you are moving and yet at the same time completely still, completely still as you fix your eyes upon this cloud that remains in constant view, knowing that there are other clouds in other places that are in constant view as well, appearing completely still. And now a soft, still, calm feeling steals down inside and you find you may absorb this feeling, just like a soft absorbent cloud within you that soaks up the feeling, saturating your very being with this comforting, floating, calm, deeply relaxing sensation. As you let go, you realize this is everywhere.

To provide a simple example to illustrate the categories of data in our thinking processes, consider a person who wants to travel from her home to a different city. With nominal data, she would likely form the conviction that she must use a particular road from home to this other city. Now her options are restricted. If the road is blocked she is stuck, with no alternatives.

But when this same woman decides she just wants to reach this other city, she then becomes aware of alternative routes to the same end. By starting with a general goal, more choices become available. Now she can choose from a variety of paths to reach this city. More than that: if she just wants to reach her destination by driving or otherwise, she can now consider alternative modes of transportation. Notice the multi-layered options that come into awareness, paths as well as means to the same goal. Use of higher awareness naturally leads to mental, emotional, and behavioral flexibility. This flexibility is one hallmark of personal well-being. In simpler terms, you could say that starting with the big picture about a situation allows greater insight and awareness of solutions. This perspective also represents a difference between micro- and macro-management.

Now let's examine the structure of a sentence in more detail. By evaluating each word in a sentence, you can identify what level of awareness the speaker is drawing from. Consider the following. A client states, "I'm always late for everything." What categories is this person utilizing in making this statement? First, we need to identify the players in this statement. Not that we're going to engage in a grammar lesson, but we do need to be aware of the crucial, meaningful parts of this statement.

Certain parts of any sentence actively display the way someone categorizes data. If you think about the subject, object, verb, adjectives, and nouns within any given sentence, you find that each represents a particular category of awareness. Yes, just about every word in a sentence represents some level of awareness. This seems true because all words ultimately stem from the pool of all words, but at each successively higher level of awareness the pool of available words expands. The result is that the words chosen to construct a sentence reveal the level of awareness, and thus the possibilities within the perceptual framework expressed in the sentence.

In the statement about being late for everything, the parts representing awareness categories include "I", "always", "late", and "everything". This actually then provides four opportunities for intervention. Let's look at each of these elements, one at a time, taking it through the full continuum of awareness.

By using the personal pronoun "I", a singular person is selected from the whole population and also from the huge number of various categories contained within the population. To which aspect of his I, or self, is he referring? What aspects-qualities of his I is he leaving out? The word "always" functions as a behavioral measurement, since always implies various ways of showing up late in the all-nothing category of always late. The only alternative to the nominal "always late" would be represented as never late. The word "late" is a category on a time continuum. Utilizing the time continuum to consider other possible scenarios can loosen perception. The use of the word "everything" is another all-nothing category regarding the events in his life. Surely exceptions exist to this everything belief.

We could create a sort of "awareness expander" with words. Before you expressed anything like the following, though, you would need to be sure to have established rapport and a trusting relationship with your client so that he would know how to receive and interpret your words. Also, offer this particular pattern in a tongue-in-cheek style or one of wry wit.

Addressing the belief that one is always late for everything might sound like this:

> So you think that you are always late for everything? Well, just what is late? I mean, is it 5 seconds, 5 minutes, 14 minutes, or 38 minutes? Is on time only the precise fleeting second when you said you'd be there? But then you might end up generously saying that anything that is the exact fleeting second of the designated arrival time *and anything earlier* is considered on time. However, what about those folks that have this need to be early, I mean really early, like 20 to 30 minutes early? Then there are those folks that camp out somewhere, perhaps two to three days in advance, to get tickets for some big event. And are you the only one who is ever late? Aren't there degrees of lateness and varying numbers of people who are late? Do you know some people who may be late sometimes and other people who are even later than you are? Are these people late for being late? Further, I bet you're always on time to go to the bathroom, at least since you learned how. [*The last sentence is optional; to be used only if you know enough about the person to be sure it won't offend. The purpose is to connect this individual to at least one process in which he recognizes and complies with a good sense of timing.*]

Once we strip away the presented concern, we may actually get down to the real issue this person wants to resolve that manifests itself in tardiness. Notice how we simply apply a stretch to awareness, expanding the category to include more possibilities.

The following offers a practical example of these categories of data or the continuum of awareness. It is drawn from the case of a client I worked with in the past. A woman, we'll call her Susan, came in for counseling because she was struggling with a limiting conviction that "everybody tells me it (her life) will never work." Each word in this sentence, with the possible exception of "will", represents some category of data and thus a perceptual level and resultant style of thinking. Yet even the word "will" represents a nominal point of view. "Will" suggests certainty rather than possibility. If we substitute the word might or could, we open up more uncertainty about the believed outcome—and thus at least an ordinal, if not an interval perspective, as other possibilities are considered.

We explored various aspects of this woman's beliefs, style of living, and general history. In collecting details, she cited five people who had consistently put her down, including her mother who is now deceased, rendering maternal pronouncements part of the dead hand of the past. Once Susan described the sources of her distress and began experiencing the sadness associated with this limiting belief, I analyzed her language pattern to help her shift awareness.

To address this limiting belief, I said:

> This everybody collection that so consistently tells you every time that it will never work—your life, not theirs—may lead you to think you're no good. But what if these words are not sound? Just who is this everybody anyway, five people? How many of the Chinese are in on this opinion? What about the Russians and people living in the Middle East, not to mention your next door neighbor or the other people living in your town, your county, your state, and your country? So this group of five [*at this point I hold up five fingers on one hand*] that you think speaks for everyone actually leaves out a billion or so people. These five represent a billion or more? *Everybody [emphasizing the five fingers]…always…tells me it will never work out!*

At this point Susan begins laughing out loud and I repeat the final statement again, very slowly and deliberately. After I finish, she responds, "Now I can't think about that [*her belief*] without laughing." Susan went on to identify a more realistic and resourceful belief that allowed her to embrace the parts of her life that she felt were satisfying and to build on these for future satisfaction.

Below I identify several questions to consider when working with clients. These questions can help you identify the level of awareness represented by the client's words and lead to identifying opportunities for expanding the client's awareness.

Theme: Identifying how someone categorizes the information or data presented.

Questions to ask:

1. What are the personal pronoun and data chunk size variables within the person's statement?
2. What category of data does the current statement exemplify?

3. What labels are used and to whom or what are they applied?
4. What would be a statement fitting into the next lower category of data? For example, if an individual displays ordinal data, what would a nominal data statement about the same information sound like?
5. If the person makes a ordinal statement, how would an interval statement sound?
6. What would a statement about the same information sound like using the ratio category of data?
7. What new perceptions come into view using larger categories of data?
8. What potential solutions can now be recognized?
9. What effect could such new statements and awareness have on the underlying limiting beliefs of a client and what might a new belief sound like?

Additional question: Is perfectionism the superimposition of nominal data on an otherwise naturally existing range of achievement levels? Perfectionism presupposes an end point exists for any given category and that this end point can be reached. It seems that perfectionism attempts to impose nominal data upon ratio data. They just won't fit. But a perfectionist presupposes they do or will fit, thus driving himself into a frenzy trying to make this happen. Presuppositions can restrict us or free us to varying degrees, depending on the size of the frame presented within the presupposition.

Chapter 2
Gestalt Categories of Framing

This next section presents the second tier that makes up our information-processing system. The second tier consists of how we go about organizing the information within our awareness into a meaningful whole. We tend to treat stimuli that come into our awareness as separate from the larger, all-inclusive whole of existing information. We then process this segregated information by identifying parts and assembling them into some meaningful whole. This second tier, then, involves the early stage of creating meaning as we link various items to form a subset of the whole. The principles of perception identified by Gestalt psychology serve as a way of describing this second-tier processing.

Gestalt psychology's roots trace back to the late 1800s in Germany. Loosely translated, gestalt, means "whole" or "form", as in something taking form within the mind and making "sense". The branch of psychology known as Gestalt (Wertheimer, 1912) focused on how we detect meaning in our environment. In the process of studying perception, Gestalt psychology came to identify seven dynamic elements that combine to help us create forms or wholes within our environment. Below is a list and description of these Gestalt elements, as well as an account of how they are manifested in daily life.

Gestalt Perceptual Categories
I. Proximity

Items tend to become associated with each other if they exist near each other in time or space. Original work with perception and proximity involved visual items. For example, people were shown items grouped in various ways on a sheet of paper. Researchers found that people looking at these items tended to consider items as belonging to the same group if they were closer together than the rest of the items as a group.

Notice the lines in Figure 2:1. In the first group, presupposing you see three sets of eight lines due to spacing, these first eight lines appear as a single group since they exist in close proximity. In the second set of lines we see what might be observed as two sets of four lines. If the gap between the first set of four and the second set were smaller, you would likely decide the two sets were a single set of eight lines. In the third set, you see what appear to be four groups of two lines each. The spacing between the lines tends to set them off as separate groups. The closeness or distance between items, proximity, usually leads to natural grouping.

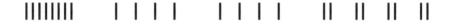

Figure 2.1: *Gestalt Grouping*

The meaning of proximity in time may be rather obvious, a set time frame. But space proximity can be trickier to understand. For the purposes of this work, we will consider spatial proximity to include physical space as well as situations and events. So space proximity includes the room in which a conflict occurs between two or more people and the particular events taking place within the space.

In a marital relationship, you could delimit a conflict narrowly using time and space and conclude that this marriage was quite conflicted. But if the frame of time and space (events) were to be expanded, you would probably find that experience included harmony and happiness as well. This inclusion of other information leads to a different perspective on the relationship.

Proximity plays a crucial role in meaning making. Proximity establishes a frame in time and space, determining the elements available for making meaning of any given event. This frame sections off a small area of time and space. Within this frame are found the items we use to make sense of an experience. We restrict the range of time and space through utilizing the principle of proximity. I suspect that the more traumatic the event an individual experiences, the smaller the temporal and spatial frame used to determine the meaning of that event.

Once again, we find another example of the continuum of awareness and its influence. If the continuum expands, the traumatized person can consider times when they experienced safety. By expanding the spatial element, they can become aware of situations-settings in which they experienced safety. Often expanding awareness is the foundation for treating and resolving post-traumatic syndromes.

The case of Carol illustrates proximity at work in limiting awareness, leading to trauma-driven limiting beliefs. Carol grew up in a home with an alcoholic father who was prone to violent outbursts. One particular incident Carol remembers when she was five years old took place in the dining room, while the family ate dinner. Without warning, her very drunken father exploded in rage, reaching out with his open hand and striking Carol in the face. She was thrown from her chair onto the floor. She had no idea of any offense that might have prompted her father's rage, if indeed she had committed any offense.

Proximity led Carol to attempt to make sense of this event using the information available right there and then, at the "scene of the crime". In this scene, temporal proximity included only the few seconds just before, during, and immediately after the event. The meaning that Carol derived from this unforeseen blow was that she was a "bad girl". When we utilize proximity and then bring in egocentricity and transductive logic (discussed in the next section), we come to believe that we are the cause of events that occur in a tiny microcosm.

Space proximity might be restricted to noticing the interaction between Carol and her father. This proximity frame excludes other people in the room, as well as other actions by her father over time and in different spaces before, during, and after the event. Notice how expanding the frame over time and space admits more diverse information. Even if just a few examples exist of the offender treating her differently, many other examples come to light of other people treating her in a much different manner. Such diversity of information creates useful cognitive dissonance. This dissonance makes it more difficult for the limiting belief formed within narrow margins of proximity to hold together. By expanding the space taken into account, additional information comes to light. The gestalt frame then begins to wobble and soon falls apart, as too many examples running contrary to the current belief or explanation come to be known. The old belief, or gestalt, can no longer hold because a greater space has been opened up and divergent factors coexist within this space.

The use of proximity can mislead us in many ways. While we may think the event within the proximity frame begins and ends there, more likely the event in the proximity frame has roots extending a long way back in time and space. Just as words represent the expression or projection of thoughts, emotions, and beliefs, any given action represents the culmination of an indeterminate period in time and space. Usually the ingredients focused upon within a narrowly proximate frame were the least influential in prompting the outcome. In other words, the supposed precipitating events "causing" some outcome often contribute little to it; they are just the most recent and therefore noticeable elements, because we rely on proximity.

Items within the immediate vicinity tend only to correlate with, not to cause, the scrutinized event. As a brief hypnotic statement designed to stimulate thought about both past and present and hinting at the future, consider the following: "Now is a byproduct of before. How long before...you know this, realizing now and the possibilities?"

Here is a simple example of hypnotic language addressing proximity:

> Take a moment to think about a time when you felt in a better mood than you do now, searching through your memories to find an example of when you felt better, knowing that when you find the first example, you find more and more...better examples until you find several that are better and bigger. Savor the feeling you have as you

step into this fully. Maybe it was from your past or maybe it is from your future that you have yet to experience and want to, knowing you will now.

What makes the language pattern above an example of proximity in action? If you followed and responded to the language, you opened and searched through a file in your mind labeled better mood or good mood. Once you opened the file, you found similar examples of the theme, feeling better or feeling good. These examples in your memory are stored together in close *proximity*, since they are alike.

How can you address proximity that involves an emotionally distressing event? Generally you can extend time and space outward from what was the original proximity frame around this emotionally distressing event. In the distressing event, there exist some kind of victim and offender. In stretching out time and space beyond the initial proximity frame, consider the following words:

> Notice the different features of the offender over time and space, then those of other individuals, their varied behaviors, different settings, and the many different types of people, moods, behaviors, and settings, along with varied tasks, goals, and outcomes. Notice also how the offender has a timeline and how he changes as he grows younger and smaller. Notice what events in his life indicate the early threads of the eventual action. Notice how many events in the main character's life from day to day and year to year before had absolutely nothing to do with you; rather he was amassing a storehouse of negative energy.

By working through time and space, you create the means of loosening linear thinking, finding possible solutions. At some point in a resolution, some aspect of the supposed problem's structure is reversed or looked at in the opposite way, inverted. Rather than the victim supposedly contributing to the offender's action, we find that the obverse is true. The offender's pre-existing state contributed to the victim's reaction. This can liberate the victim from erroneously believing they caused the aggressor's action.

How do you go about choosing whether to address perceptions or states when working with clients? If someone shows an apparently strong need for the state, such that it seems a necessary defense mechanism, consider first addressing their perceptions or available information by expanding awareness. Expanding awareness will inevitably lead to information contrary to current beliefs and state of being. A cognitive dissonance will occur. You can then let the client's processing of new information bring about change within the client's personality. If someone does not seem strongly committed to their state, then consider directly addressing it, allowing the corresponding shifts in perception naturally to bring different information to consciousness.

I offer the following brief language pattern addressing temporal proximity:

> Sometimes you want to interpret your present through your past and sometimes you want to interpret your past through your present. Since the reverse holds true at times, the solution is to use whichever works better—you'll know by how it feels.

II. Figure-Ground

Figure-ground means dividing a larger perceived chunk into both foreground and background. This equates to what you pay attention to versus what you ignore. Your figure provides the material from which you form beliefs. Change your figure and change your belief—go figure.

This category determines what the individual focuses on, what makes up their figure. In order to decide on a figure, you also have to make a ground. The ground is what the individual ignores but this ground is fertile in rich resources that can provide a solution. The ground may be in the moment or may stretch out over time. You could also think of the figure as being the conscious mind, while the ground represents the unconscious mind. What does an individual notice about self, others, life, and the environment? Now notice a dichotomy. This may be an outline of two parts within that which have split: a good self–bad self split. Utilizing the process of figure-ground splits an otherwise intact whole into two separate parts.

You may have noticed how figure-ground is similar to centering. The difference is that centering happens for about the first seven years of life. Making figure-ground distinctions recurs throughout a lifetime. Centering essentially makes no reference to the rest of the whole, while figure requires a ground to exist as a figure.

The following is an example of a hypnotic language pattern involving figure-ground in response to a client's presented concern about losing people in his life about whom he cared:

> As you sit here wondering and worrying about who left you, and wondering how they could leave you if you cared for them, you may then wonder how dangerous it is to care. But it may be more important to notice whom you have found, not lost, and what you gained from whom you found. Noticing this permanent gain you received from each person accumulating and recognizing that, while this experience carries over time, it was made up of unique experiences with each—each experience being the one and only one you will ever have, one of a kind—is important. Each second is unique, like diamonds from a mine, except they are yours to keep and collect. Immerse yourself in this uniqueness and cherish what you find. Cherish this one of a kind jewel in a unique way, holding it and yet looking forward to the next unique one to add to your cherished collection of gems, so that you move from treasure to treasure, never forgetting, always remembering, and eagerly looking forward to the next new one you knew, you know, you will know … and the sharing.

Theme: Similar to centering, looking for the focus.

Questions to ask:

1. What part of the whole is this person's focus? The whole means the infinite, all. From this whole, an individual selects some general part but then narrows the focus this much more. He may focus on his father. But what aspects of his father comprise his focus? (When you search for the whole from which the person selects the figure, you begin to observe solutions that you can introduce later.)
2. What is being ignored from the category "father" in this example, and from the larger whole of all relationships (other relationships of his and relationships of others in general)? This rich material, counter or alternative examples, often provides the content of hypnotic language.

III. Similarity

Similarity means noticing items in the environment of a similar theme. Have you ever noticed that when you get a new car, brand new, or just new to you, that suddenly it seems that this is the only car you see on the road? It seems to be everywhere.

Also, homonyms, words with a similar sound, fit nicely within this category and lend themselves well to hypnotic language.

In order to perpetuate a problem or belief, one must sort for similarities. These identified similarities may be examples of current experiences that validate a belief or may be anticipatory elements in a future environment that will substantiate an existing belief. If someone focuses on solutions, certain items will be found. But if one limits oneself in response to a past trauma, the tendency is to sort for items in the current environment similar to the environment at the time of the trauma, thus finding only reasons to remain afraid.

Sorting for similarities maintains a trance, while sorting for differences breaks a trance, providing new choices. I would suggest that one trait of genius is its ability to go "a-categorical," into an absence of categories, separating each item from every other so that any item can fit anywhere, creating infinite possibilities, permitting combining items in more resourceful ways.

Even if a person sorting for dangerous stimuli does not find these dreaded items, in severe cases, they will assume that these items *will* turn up at some point, acting *as if* these items were present *now*. The deepest intent of this scanning process would seem to be to gain a sense of safety. But scanning for potential danger and acting as if these dangers are here and now actually brings a sense of fear. Notice how the imagination can function as a limiting device or as the source of solutions, depending on what we imagine.

The Gestalt concept of similarities is all about categories. What feature of an observed item do we use to represent the whole? To categorize we choose a figure from the ground, and then sort for similar figures on different grounds across different times and situations. We then are tempted to string together these supposedly similar events to arrive at a "conclusion". To render this more concrete: the new car we buy then makes us more aware of this and similar cars, becoming our focus and leading us to find only more of the same. And nothing ever changes, does it? Sorting for similarities tells us this is true.

Using hypnotic language to address similarities may utilize a focus on differences to help expand awareness of resources and options. The following example illustrates sorting for similarities versus differences when working with a client experiencing chronic physical pain. Tony, we'll call him, described frequent episodes of not being able to hold things in his hands properly. He reported that he often dropped things such as kitchen utensils or glasses and other small handheld items. He came to believe that his inability to hold things in his hands meant he was losing his mind. He had come to pay attention only to the times he dropped things and he wove these together into a gestalt, to feeling as though this was all he did, which meant he was "going crazy".

To counter his illogical reasoning, I declared:

> Tony, I know that you feel as though you are dropping everything you touch. But it may be that this is all you're noticing. Have you ever bought a car, a new car, or just one that's new to you? And as soon as you started on the road to go home you began to notice just how many people had this kind of car. You noticed this more and more until it seemed this was the only kind of car on the road. [*He nodded in agreement.*] So it may turn out that, just as you didn't notice the cars you didn't observe on the road, there may be many more cars that are different, not similar. So too it may almost certainly be true that you hold onto many more things than you drop. Think about an average day and just how many things you pick up and how long you hold them. Notice how much you pick up and how long you hold it; just what percentage of the time is this true?

From here we found a way to sort over time, past, present, and future, to derive new meaning from the majority of incidents when he held onto things rather than the minority of incidents when he dropped them. He now had a new similarity to sort for and could find evidence of a different sort that reassured him of his well-being.

We will revisit the case of Tony in more detail in the Chapter Five.

Theme: Look for common themes or threads in an individual's perceptions.

Questions to ask:

1. Utilizing a sort of timeline approach, what theme or common thread does this person reveal to you through the habitual focus from situation to situation?
2. What items do they sort for?
3. What beliefs does this sorting style suggest are held about self, life, or others?

Notice how similarities fit in with figure-ground and the later category of continuation to filter in and filter out certain information that maintains the status quo.

IV. Closure

Closure means completing an item perceived to be unfinished, filling in the missing feature that permits a sense of closure. When used poorly, this can lead to jumping to conclusions. Inductive logic enables one to note that closure is similar to inductive logic. Inductive logic makes generalizations beyond a specific example while closure arrives at conclusions on a case-by-case basis. Impulsive and impatient people often over-use closure and end up blocking out alternative information and solutions. People also predict their future using closure.

Closure is a key principle in hypnotic language. Gaps in perception invite listener participation. Leaving gaps in words or meanings for the listener to fill in forms a foundation of hypnotic language. Closure is what the client uses to fill in the details within vague communications made by the therapist. Clients tailor general information to their own needs.

When a person engages in the process of closure it may be need-driven. We tend to fill in blanks according to need. If you challenge perceptions, you really challenge the need, so acknowledge the perception, but then notice and address the need, not the perception. If you only challenge the perception, you may stir up only a client's defenses.

An example of perception and need interacting, not closure, was offered when I worked with a woman who wanted to stop smoking. As we moved deeper into her rationale for the purpose served by smoking, we found that she smoked in order to feel calm. Serenity then was her need. But had I just focused on the perception that smoking was a harmful behavior to motivate quitting, a tug-of-war would have ensued that would likely have manifested itself as client resistance. What it would really mean was that I had not addressed the underlying need that was driving the whole process. Once we addressed her need to experience calm and identified alternative ways of experiencing this without detriment, she was able to give up smoking.

As an example of closure in action, notice when someone uses the word "almost". This word invites us to convert an *almost* experience into an actual experience. One closes the gap between what was *almost* a problem and an actual problem into an anxiety-provoking experience, as if the event had really happened. Now there is a problem but the act of closure is the problem, not any actual external event. Helping focus on the gap between *did* and *did not* can be a source of great relief.

Pessimism needs closure in order to remain active. Someone sunk in pessimism must predict a negative outcome and then believe it not only *will* come true but that it is *already* true. This robs one of motivation. To one pessimistic client who based her negative predictions about her future on biased memories from her past, I said, "How does feeling bad keep you from feeling bad?" This simple line addressed both the process and the need driving the process; as a result, she began to notice how her closure was counterproductive to her stated goal of experiencing happiness. I went on to say to this client:

> How many times did you think you knew what was going to happen, but you didn't? And how many times have you not waited for all the information to come in and just assumed you knew, but you didn't? But this does not mean you will fill in the blanks in your future in your

present, does it? And since you really want to make the best and most informed decision possible, you'd want to allow yourself to remain open to receiving valuable information. Now won't you…gain from this?

Theme: Identify what is missing and how someone responds to missing information.

Questions to ask:

1. What missing pieces of information about a given situation does this person fill in through applying imagination rather than facts?
2. How does such "fact" creation play out over time regarding past conclusions with insufficient evidence, as well as in predictions about the future with no evidence?
3. Closure means that an individual is no longer open to possibilities. They have made up their mind, formed a belief, and cling to this belief. What is this belief?

A crucial question: What information must be ignored to maintain the belief in question?

V. Simplicity

Simplicity entails reducing elements perceived to the simplest form. In courting simplicity, the least cognitive effort possible is used to interpret the information received, ignoring details that make differences. And the difference is the difference. Simplicity is responsible for entrenched prejudices. For example, all tall people are clumsy; the Irish drink too much; and people with red hair have bad tempers.

Through simplicity, we may try a shortcut that leads to twice as much work. Simplicity is at work when we decide it is too much effort to change our beliefs about something. Simplicity is maintained by ignoring exceptions to a self-declared rule. We'll just leave our old belief the same old way it was and ignore the train coming down the track at us. Don't confuse me with the facts; I've already made up my mind. Words such as "bad" simplify the concept of harmful; words such as "good" simplify the concept of beneficial. Hypnotic language utilizes simplified words, which is good—you can decide how.

Simplicity in conversation often includes using general, catch-all terms rather than specific terms. Using such general terms one oversimplifies and then includes too much information in a particular category rather than discriminate essential from inessential details. Simplicity sticks with general information, leaving out details that would alter how information is categorized. Closure and continuation seal the deal with simplicity.

Simplicity in action leads to someone saying, "Oh, what's the use? It's all the same anyway and I can't figure it (a task) out anyway." Using hypnotic language, you might respond:

> I know that you believe that this job will never work out because you're thinking about the times it did not, noticing particulars that could make a particularly big difference. And you say it's just easier to give up and continue believing this won't work to keep it simple, a one-size-fits-all formula. But this approach really complicates life, doesn't it? If you didn't adopt this stance you'd be feeling better. How much simpler is it really to feel bad every time you think and believe this, instead of making different choices that lead to simply feeling better? I know you only say what you said because what you most want is a solution that will work better—isn't that so?

In a significant relationship, one party does not speak when things go wrong for them. This choice is supposedly simpler than experiencing conflict. But, as you know, this "simpler" choice sets up a bigger, more complicated problem that expands and becomes multilayered. And, if it really is simpler not to speak up, then why don't you feel better, and why don't good things follow your self-suppression?

Theme: Identify ways in which someone overlooks or distorts information in order to ignore potentially belief-altering details.

Questions to ask:

1. Consider not only what the person is ignoring but also how it is ignored. What do they pay attention to (figure) instead?

2. How is contrary information handled? For example, does this individual form a "belief dumpster," a sort of excusing or rationalizing of exceptions to their rule so they can dispose of them wholesale?
3. What issues or fears may arise when you look more deeply into these exceptions?
4. What beliefs do they then expose?

This leads to the next category, known as cognitive dissonance reduction.

VI. Cognitive Dissonance Reduction

Cognitive Dissonance Reduction refers to the need to reconcile disparate perceptions and beliefs either by changing perceptions or beliefs. When you experience something contrary to what you believe, you distort or generalize the experience, or you retain the experience and modify your belief. Sometimes we invoke simplicity, ignoring details, to retain an old belief in the face of evidence to the contrary. Changing beliefs leads to other changes; somehow, we think it's simpler to maintain an old belief.

Consider the term "overachiever" to illustrate dissonance reduction. Maybe you know someone whom others consider to be an overachiever. This notion of acting as an overachiever has two parts: actual performance and beliefs about capability. But whose belief: that of the individual or of those observing? Can anyone really overachieve, going beyond what they are able to achieve? It seems that if we perform at a particular level, then we are able, or we could not have attained this level. But some people, hearing they are overachievers, soft-pedal their performance to bring it back in line with expectations or past performance levels. It may be more accurate to say that overachieving is actually due to low expectations on the part of the expectant, whether observer or performer. We seem to have a tendency to behave in line with our expectations; it may benefit us at least to suspend expectations so we do not so easily fall prey to this temptation to gain dissonance reduction by reducing performance quality.

An example of hypnotic language addressing dissonance reduction was elicited by a client describing an internal conflict between what she believed she wanted to do and what her husband told her she should do. You respond by saying:

> It sure can feel very confusing and frustrating not knowing which choice to make and wanting to make everybody happy. But consider that these wants and shoulds come from two very different places, one in you and the other outside of you. One choice feels right to you, it fits just like the shoes you're wearing today; they fit your feet and circumstances. The other feels wrong, yet disappointing others troubles you. So really your concern is less what to do than what to do about the other person's disappointment. And you really have nothing to do with another's disappointment because you do not and cannot cause it. If you did, you could make it disappear regardless of the choice you make. So it may be confusing but this will clear when you make the choice you can control instead of courting a cascade of confusing frustrations that will occur otherwise that you cannot control. But you know this, or you would not be sitting here with me today, telling yourself you know, you know?

Theme: Identify discrepancies between beliefs held and realistic evidence.

Questions to ask:

1. This standoff between perceptions and beliefs carries much weight. Identify the two opposing forces at work. What perceptions and beliefs are at odds?
2. Is either of the sides, belief or perception, tied to a more powerful belief or perception operating under the conscious mind's surface conflict, actually driving the choices of the individual? If so, what might this person believe or perceive that "holds together" the presented issue? This belief may exist as something an individual is trying to prevent from becoming a reality (failure), or fears may become a reality (success). Notice how belief tends to drive perception and perception, in turn, tends to lend support for belief.
3. What will happen when either the belief or the perception changes? What will then become the battleground—a deeper belief or perception that may actually represent the original conflict?

VII. Continuation

Continuation means maintaining a particular perception or mind-set beyond the original point of perception. Continuation in perception compares to the old Newtonian law that states that a body in motion tends to stay in motion, while a body at rest tends to stay at rest. When some people get angry, they often even get mad at someone who tries to cheer them up, continuing the madness. Continuation resembles a trance state. The hard part is coming out of the trances we go through in daily living. Stop continuation and start change. Think of habit when thinking of continuation, since continuing tends to become a habit. Continuation is also part of why you may have to ask a person the same question two or three times in order to loosen their grip on whatever focus they are maintaining. We even tend to engage in what might be thought of as physical continuation. Have you ever been on a boat or sea cruise? How long after you got on dry land did you *continue* to feel as if you were still on the water? Note how, once we perceive in a particular way, we tend to continue in this same mode of perception.

Notice how continuation and dissonance reduction function hand in hand. Continuation is allowed to continue, whilst reducing dissonance eliminates disparate information that would have necessitated a change in beliefs. For example, when a person with low self-esteem chooses relationships, they often select those who will help them maintain their low self-esteem. They become so accustomed to poor treatment that, when someone suddenly comes along and treats them well, inquires about their well-being, and encourages them, they suspect the motives of this unusual person. Reducing dissonance invites them to continue in the same old beliefs and to dismiss the newcomer.

Continuation appears in the client's story to you when they describe habitual responses or longstanding beliefs. Often, a client comes to see a counselor because they are maintaining some undesirable, self-defeating system of beliefs, emotions, and behaviors. Continuing can appear like an addiction, an addiction to a way of life in the face of evidence showing that this way of life is harming the individual. No doubt some unconscious need or deficit is driving this process in an attempt somehow to satisfy this felt deficit, but it only does more harm.

Another example of hypnotic language addressing continuation was inspired by a woman who tended to defer to others when making decisions. She habitually deferred to others and then suffered emotionally as a result of shortchanging herself. Observing this, I said:

> It can be difficult knowing what to do and old decision-making styles can become so habitual that you don't know you used them until you feel frustrated and angry afterwards. Knowing how to know what you really want and need would be very useful. Just how do you and how does anyone really know what they want and need? In some homes, a family member may open up the refrigerator, take out an item— milk for example—and smell it. They might make a strange face and then ask the family-designated checker to smell the milk to decide if it has gone bad. If it has, they throw it out.

The client nodded and said that she is her family's designated food checker. I continued, "So you know how to do this, but just how do you know that you know what you know?" She paused, searched inside herself, and then answered, "I just use what I know!"

We then went on to clarify this internal knowing and then just left it...trusting that she would know when and how to rely on this internal sense of knowing to stop old, self-damaging habits. Follow-up in several weeks revealed that she had made numerous lifestyle changes affecting herself and her entire family system for the better.

Theme: Look for patterns of beliefs, states, or behaviors occurring across situations that contribute to the client's overall problem.

Questions to ask:

1. What specific behaviors, states, or beliefs seem to have a life of their own, so that they continue whatever this person does, contributing to the problem?
2. How does continuing this style contribute to the problem or keep the problem alive?
3. Where or when does this individual continue in their behavior-state consistently, and where or when do they not do this?
4. How is this person utilizing their figure or focus, selecting similar figures, enabling them to continue a pattern?

Notice how each of these Gestalt perceptual styles lends support to the other, holding a perception in place. If you change any one of these elements, the whole, or gestalt, changes. These Gestalt perceptual styles make up the boundaries of frames.

Chapter 3
Cognitive Styles Identified by Piaget

This section presents the third tier of the four-tier information-processing system. In *Hypnotic Language: Its Structure and Use* (Burton and Bodenhamer, 2000) the work of Jean Piaget was drawn on extensively. Piaget's groundbreaking work, refined by research that followed, revealed the cognitive styles that children use in processing information in their world. These same cognitive styles prominent in childhood are also used by adults at times. It seems that personal trauma experienced in childhood increases the likelihood of utilizing the cognitive styles of childhood.

These thinking styles also often surface during times of emotional intensity in adulthood, without prior emotional trauma. It appears that our mental focus narrows, perhaps instinctively, during times of emotional intensity. Maybe at some level this serves as a self-preservation mechanism. Regardless of the potential benefits at certain times, the cognitive processing styles that are inevitable in childhood play a significant role in the structure of personal problems. The inverse of these cognitive processes, expanding awareness, plays a significant role in solving personal problems. As you will see, hypnotic language addresses and reverses limiting styles of thinking.

Below is a list and description of cognitive styles, followed by a series of questions that you can ask of your clients that may help further elicit the presence of a cognitive style and its influence in a client's problem. Each cognitive style listed will also be explained using a case example. This information lends personal meaning to the ingredients selected by the client from the whole environment by our Gestalt perceptual styles.

The purpose of providing such cognitive information is that these thinking styles influence us mentally and emotionally, not only in childhood, but at various times in our life span. These thinking styles seem to exist primarily, if not exclusively, at the nominal level of awareness. Further, these thinking styles tend to form the internal, cognitive foundation of our personal problems at any time in our lives. Hypnotic language speaks to these thinking styles, seeking to help clients move beyond this style to more resourceful ways of thinking that permit solutions to be discovered and implemented.

As we progress through this work, note how hypnotic language scripts utilize words and sentence structure that naturally adopt the same linguistic style that the client used in creating his or her problem. To some degree, hypnotic language relies on client thinking in the styles identified by Piaget both to address the cognitive structure of the problem and to bring about change.

I. Egocentrism

Egocentrism means believing that what you think or feel is true for everyone. If a child needs new shoes, they think that everyone needs new shoes. A person displaying egocentricity can only see things from their point of view. The world revolves around them. They lack empathy. If an egocentric adult thinks or feels something, they think that everyone either thinks or *should* think this. Self-centered is a synonym for egocentric. Egocentricity also results in someone taking events around him personally. Everything is about you, since you are the center of the world. We all harbor degrees of egocentricity. It depends on how you use it. Egocentricity is the selfish cousin of empathy. While empathy puts you in others' shoes, egocentricity puts others in your shoes.

Egocentricity also sets up many faulty presuppositions. Once we decide some situation is about us, we then activate resources to direct the outcome so as to make us feel safe or good in some sense. Since we *presuppose* the situation revolves around us, we then must steer it and those involved according to our best interests.

At the same time, egocentricity can become an ally of hypnotic language. The client receiving hypnotic language naturally applies the language to self. They thereby internally apply the healing concepts carried by words to their problematic issues, integrating new information and thus transforming the old. How does anti-inflammatory medication know where to go within the body? Well, it isn't really localized but it affects the area needing change, bringing it into line with the rest of the self.

Egocentricity appears to be the glue or catalyst for other Piagetian categories. Egocentricity views life as a set of adversarial relationships, inviting defensiveness. If you stop egocentricity, then other categories lose their incentive force and no longer need to be adopted.

How Egocentricity Sounds in Conversation

When a client uses "I" statements, you can be sure some degree of egocentricity lurks behind this. What is not meant here is the kind of appropriate "I" statement that takes responsibility for the self. Egocentric statements manifest emotional distress or self-praise in content and process. And when someone attributes their own distress to someone else, egocentricity has a hand in this, too. Expecting certain things of others may also stem from egocentricity.

I want to briefly step aside to identify a slight variation in the way egocentricity presents itself. This other form of egocentricity is subtler and may appear as a sort of codependency. Here, someone tries to please or placate others because they think other people's actions and moods concern them. We tend to display one of two general responses when egocentricity dominates us. Either we try to orchestrate the situation and the people in it to our best advantage, or we try to please everyone in order to appear in the best possible light. The second method is a different kind of orchestration. Have you ever noticed how sometimes a dating or married couple will include each of these versions of egocentricity, the manipulator and the pleaser working in concert as complementary versions of the same dynamic?

It should be added that when someone states they are angry at someone, this anger is often, in part, anger at the self for a decision that occurred *before* the other's supposedly offensive act. Expressed anger at another person is in response to offensive behavior by another. But if we step back in time, some decision was likely made by the offended individual before the actual event, setting him or her up as a victim. I do not refer to victims of crime, who are innocent people who were at the wrong place at the wrong time.

One additional note about felt anger: Our anger may actually exist about our self-limiting perception and self-limiting beliefs. But in the heat of the moment we tend to look outside of self for the source of our felt anger. If we first look within and examine how we may be limiting our self through narrow awareness or restricting beliefs we may empower our self. We may then extract our self from restrictions, freeing our self from anger thereby opening our self to constructive solutions.

As an illustration, consider the example of Anita and her husband Sam. The type of victimization that I'm referring to results from an ongoing relationship whereby Anita continues to put herself in a subordinate position to Sam, who then takes advantage of her. Anita reports anger at Sam, with good reason. But useful, change-promoting anger would be better aimed at Anita's prior decision that placed her in the position of being disrespected, when she knew full well how such a situation would unfold. Once this decision is accessed, if she can move beyond egocentricity, positive change may occur.

You may ask how egocentricity is involved in Anita's decision. As an example, Anita may wish to visit an ailing relative out of town. Her husband Sam says he thinks this is a bad idea, as Anita needs her rest and the trip would be exhausting. Anita then drops her own desire and refrains from making the trip out of town. She experiences anger at Sam who, she believes, has blocked her from doing what she really wanted to do.

Egocentricity displays itself in Anita's belief that, if she goes against Sam's wishes, he will be upset with her. She then believes that she is *causing* Sam's distress. But actually she is causing her own distress by not honoring her own wishes. Her belief that she causes Sam's feelings and that she is responsible for peace at home stems from egocentricity. Egocentricity tells Anita that she is the center of the world, not in a selfish but in a co-dependent way: she holds herself responsible for all that others experience. Anita believes that because she is responsible for another's quality of life, she must conform to that person's wishes and needs.

One way of addressing the sort of anger shown in this case is to access events before the reported conflict. The dynamics revealed can provide a rich resource for reversing the problem and finding a solution. To offer another example, if Sarah wants to act assertively with her mother but fears being rude, Sarah may fret and fear rejection, feeling guilty even before confronting her mother. But a more complete picture of the dynamics of their relationship over time reveals that Sarah's mother treats her rudely at the outset of most interactions.

Once you have assessed these dynamics, you might say to Sarah something like this:

> Sarah, I realize you don't feel comfortable standing up for yourself to your mother and fear you will be rude. But your mother has already been rude to you when she put you down and called you cruel names. She is the one behaving aggressively and disrespecting you. What you are doing by standing up for yourself is just respecting yourself by not tolerating her disrespect. So really all you are doing is disrespecting her disrespect of you, so you can respect yourself. Now, isn't that true?

Then elicit the new feeling that follows as a result of this awareness—self-respect and confidence for example—and assist Sarah in knowing when and how to apply this knowledge in the future. This process actually keeps the focus on egocentricity but the content and process are altered.

Egocentricity often translates into feeling guilty, since the egocentric one may take responsibility for others' chosen emotions. Here is an example of hypnotic language applied to egocentricity involving guilt:

> When you think about your guilt and feel your guilt, I know that you can even feel guilty about feeling guilty, since you want everything to be just right. And thinking about your guilt, as I know you can, you

will notice how this is really just being over-conscientious. When you get over the "over", you notice it is nothing to feel guilty about; rather you can feel very pleased that you care so much. And feeling this care, as I know you want to, you can...feel this same care very deeply now. Now I wonder how you can...allow it to encompass both yourself and the other person as you feel and express this deep caring now.

Egocentricity as a Function of the Continuum of Awareness

For the sake of illustrating both egocentricity and the continuum of awareness in more specific terms, I will describe how egocentricity alters as it slides up the continuum. At the nominal level, as stated earlier, egocentricity manifests in a person's belief that all events that occur in life are somehow related to them. Egocentricity manifests itself in construing all events as about self, which then operates like the sun of an individual solar system made up of the people and events in their life. Events and others' actions are believed to reflect on the self. An individual may then desperately defend self, blaming others for anything and everything that goes wrong. Blaming others is the alternative to feeling one's self to be at fault. An all-or-nothing quality inheres in this way of thinking: events are either generated by the self or by others. No combination of factors or mixing of personal choices by self and various others come into consideration.

At the ordinal level of awareness, egocentricity exhibits a more flexible form of thinking, considering that somehow an event may result from a combination of one's own and others' thoughts, emotions, and behavior. Yet such thinking is still dominated by just two factors: self and others. The change is that these two factors co-exist rather than being either-or. But this ordinal level still embraces the notion that one person causes another's chosen reactions. Blame and fault-finding still frequent this level of awareness. Partly because of this duality—self and other only—one person becomes perhaps better than the other, or less or more at fault. The result is that events are still interpreted as about self, but slightly diluted by including some other person as co-contributor. The ordinal level of awareness only considers two factors, self and other. Yes, we do co-create events with others, yet how many variables from how many different sources are we influenced by and are drawn upon in this interaction? Now the possibilities expand.

At the interval level of awareness, an egocentric person can begin considering more than self and other. Degrees of one's own and others' contributions to an event now include variables outside of self-other that may have contributed to any given event. Such variables may include past events, as well as other relationships and experiences. The focus on self as the center of events diminishes considerably, dimming the need or scorekeeping. More options come to light through this interval level of awareness as broader awareness illuminates more variables and possibilities. Different response options also appear more available, as they are viewed as less about self and more about finding constructive solutions.

Further awareness expansion takes place at the ratio level. Here one reaches a whole new awareness of self, others, and events. Perceiving at the ratio level leads to realizing that each person chooses his or her own thoughts, emotions, and behaviors. Thus, another person's actions exhibit a glimpse another inner world. Another's psychic map is displayed with each expression of thought, emotion, or action. The formerly egocentric person now realizes that other people's self-expressions arise from them and are not generated externally.

Egocentricity becomes moot at this level of awareness. External stimuli become recognized as opportunities for others to project their own meanings, beliefs, and values. Self-expression is not caused by external stimuli or other people. An individual assumes responsibility for their own self-expression as accuracy of awareness and perception take into account multidimensional variables and possibilities that have existed and are current. At this level of awareness, one experiences much greater freedom, realizing that they are responsible for their own thoughts, emotions, and actions and can consider an array of options and possibilities.

Theme: Identify ways in which an individual centers a situation on self.

Questions to ask to identify egocentricity in a presenting problem:

1. How did he or she come to be at the center of this constellation, with other people and factors orbiting around him, and what necessary acts or beliefs support this process? An example is the adult child who takes responsibility for or tries to fix other family members' behavior, in particular that of a parent.
2. Around what aspects of life does this client's issue revolve, such as career, social relationships, self-esteem, etc.?
3. How does this individual come to believe the situation centers on them?
4. What limiting beliefs about self come into play as a result of this egocentricity?

II. Centration

Centration is the concept of focusing attention on only one feature of a larger whole, inducing a trance-state. Centering is the name of the process whereby you focus your awareness on a single feature of a larger whole to the exclusion of all other parts of the whole. A trance, yes? And we all do centering. The danger lies in losing sight of anything outside your centered focus and losing the ability to expand your awareness so that you can see the bigger picture. Centering also usually takes the item focused upon out of context.

You will know the client is utilizing centering because they will dwell on some cause of distress or negative belief. If you attempt to shift from this, they will come right back to focusing on this issue or this specific element. Often this focus selects behavior of her or his own, then uses this element to blame the self or forms some limiting belief. When addressing this centering, you may find it helpful first to acknowledge the *need* to focus, as the client is somehow hoping this focus on a supposed error will yield a solution—when actually, as you know, focusing on the error *is* the error.

One way to address this misguided focus is to help a client just to become aware that something outside this focus exists. You might say something like this:

It's not so much that the problem is what you're thinking, but that the solution lies in what you're not thinking. Just think about this now. And when you think about what you thought was your failure you may feel some sense of guilt over the lost opportunity to show how deeply you care. But there's no sense in this guilt when you now remember that a new opportunity to express your care exists now and you'd really hate to miss this new opportunity you know is coming up, because it's hard to say you were wrong back then, but how good does it feel to know you are right now?

To help the client enlarge awareness by including the bigger picture, you can start by acknowledging the presented problem. You can then essentially start reeling off a list of things omitted from the current focus. You can do this metaphorically as well. The focus is like noticing only one letter in the alphabet when there are 25 others. Not only are there 25 others, but there are different languages that use and combine this full complement of letters in new and different ways, not to mention other countries and ultures with these different alphabets that express many new and different ideas in new and different ways. So just what is it that you want to express, and how many different ways can you imagine yourself expressing them?

Theme: Identify an individual's focus.

Questions to ask:

1. What is the general focus of this person or their behavior?
2. Which specific features of this behavior, emotions or thoughts, does this person fixate upon?
3. What beliefs does this person derive from the practice of the centering?

III. All-or-Nothing Thinking

In extremes, the world exists as black or white, true or false. This type of thinking force fits information into one of only two categories, depriving you of essential details that need to be taken into account. The difference is the difference, making each situation and each element in it unique.

All-or-nothing thinking often appears in value statements or statements about self or beliefs that exhibit an extreme perspective. Also, in some sense, every label a person uses represents all-or-nothing thinking. Labels divide things into items that fall within a category and those that do not. Reframing provides a useful way of loosening and re-categorizing items labeled items. The idea is not to necessarily to stop all-or-nothing—though that might be desirable—but at least to make this kind of thinking work better for the client. You can also provide counter examples to the all or nothing presented, making these counter examples an extreme to really stretch and break the hold of the label.

Here is a brief example of hypnotic language that may stretch your awareness:

> When you go to the grocery store and all you want is just one item, do you ever come out with just that one item? Do you know why they put the milk at the back of the store? So that you will notice other items you may have forgotten you need. You need to remember that you really want... *these other things*. And what do you want to need? Because it's not so much that the problem is what you're thinking about, as that what you're not thinking about is the solution. Just think about that now.

In response to someone stating he believes he's a failure, you might say something like the following:

> Well, really to be a failure you'd have to fail at everything you ever tried, and do so every time, which would make you quite a successful failure. However, I find it hard to believe you fail at everything, because if you really did you'd be dead. I guess that means there are degrees of failure and that means [*"means" is needed for suggesting new meanings and a logical progression*] there are degrees of success; when you succeed in discovering this, you will begin succeeding, now. And how does this feel as you begin and continue to notice the many ways and times you succeeded, noticing just how you did this and how you felt then. Now you can again recall and do these things successfully.

You can then use the state elicited to make further progress by identifying the beliefs and perceptions accompanying this state and apply them to the issue at hand now and in the future.

Theme: Observe split perception, all-or-nothing versus a continuum.

Questions to ask:

1. How has this individual framed the problem so that only two perspectives or choices are offered? This also provides a nice opportunity to work with dialectics, opposing poles. Identify features of thoughts, emotions. and behaviors within each pole of the either/or dichotomy.
2. Something to remember: Someone adopting all-or-nothing thinking may use this perspective to come up with only two choices. This all-or-nothing may be applied to a single choice, resulting in only best- and worst-case scenarios for a single given option. The attitude is, "Well, with this choice I'll either succeed or fail miserably." (Which begs the question, how does one "succeed miserably"—but let's save this for another time.) What does the client see as the worst- and best-case scenarios for *each* of the either/or *choices* identified? Observing two extreme outcomes begins to loosen up thinking, often leading to identification of more options.
3. What crucial contrary information is left out of the all-or-nothing frame (the exceptions)?

As an afterthought, notice how egocentricity and centering necessarily contribute to an all-or-nothing point of view. The constricting perspective that stems from focusing exclusively on self or a single feature of self or environment creates rigid boundaries. The result easily mutates into either/or thinking.

IV. Irreversibility

Irreversibility denotes an inability to rewind perceptions, beliefs, or feelings to a time before the present. You cannot remember how you thought or felt or behaved before you adopted your current style because this has gone on so long it has become a habit. Strong emotions can greatly inhibit your ability to reverse course, as strong emotions tend to be "sticky." For example, when you feel angry toward someone important in your life, you tend to forget the positive characteristics they exhibited before you got mad. If you've ever heard a married couple arguing, you might have noticed that the offense that precipitates the argument seems to be held to be the offender's only behavior—all his good deeds are forgotten. Combining centering with irreversibility and all-or-nothing thinking tends to lock us into an angry mode. You may then say someone is literally stuck in anger. If you can't get past it, can you get before it?

Irreversibility may present as a sort of stasis in emotions, thoughts, or behavior. Now is all that someone may be aware of, but it is a negative, limiting now, not the larger picture over time. A lack of mental traction prevents a person from moving forward. Playing a role in this immobility is the individual's inability to recall the more highly functioning past and to invoke it in the present. Accessing past resources that proved effective then may also prove effective in the present.

Addressing irreversibility with a client who feels sad, you might say:

> You have given me a visual of what you say is your sadness. You see your sadness as a sort of embedded, buried *thing* that goes from the surface down very deep, almost all the way to the bottom. And since this sadness forms a sort of vertical timeline, such as an archeological dig might uncover, there must then exist a point underneath this sadness where it is not and where instead is some other state that existed before. Just what is this pre-existing something else that is not sadness?

The elicited state, once accessed, may prove a resource for solutions.

Theme: Explore the past for overlooked perceptions and resources.

Questions to ask:

1. How has this person lost sight of the way life was before their problem manifested itself and how they *performed effectively* prior to its appearance?
2. If life before the problem is recalled, is this memory negatively

biased by selective attention and forgetting?
3. What past resource has been forgotten that might be useful now (what has the client used effectively in the past and how did they do this)?

V. Inductive Logic

Inductive Logic is invoked when someone reaches sweeping conclusions based on a single piece of information. With runaway inductive logic you may qualify for the Olympic "conclusion jumping" team. Inductive logic, or overgeneralization, can lead to many limiting beliefs about self, based on a single or very few examples. Inductive logic encourages labeling and identity statements. Inductive logic is at work when someone believes that someone rejects them and then becomes convinced that nobody loves them or ever will. Combine inductive logic with such other categories as all-or-nothing, irreversibility, centering, and egocentric thinking, and you have a tightly knit gestalt that imprisons a person; it doesn't fit in terms of degree or accuracy of awareness. To break free, you need enlarged and enhanced awareness.

Inductive logic often expresses itself as an unspoken "therefore" implied in a value statement. Inductive logic may sound like this: "Nobody understands me." The words "nobody" and "understand" reveal the inductive logic. But underneath exists another, unspoken, inductive logic-driven statement. If nobody understands me, what does this supposedly mean? An identity statement lurks in the shadows, something like, "I'll never find anyone to love or be loved by"—or some other quantum leap without factual basis.

In response to the statement "Nobody understands me" you might say, "So this means that everybody misunderstands you?" Now you've put the client in a double bind, with no escape from rational thinking. If he says, "Well, maybe not everybody", then their inductive logic has lost its power. If, however, they respond to your statement by saying "Yes, everybody misunderstands me", then you just say, "Well, then, doesn't this just mean that I now do understand you so that it's *not* true that everybody misunderstands you?"

Theme: Look for overgeneralized conclusions.

Questions to ask:

1. What conclusions is this person drawing?
2. What labels or identity statements are being used about self, others, and life?
3. What unspoken, inductive logic-driven statement may lurk beneath the spoken one?

VI. *Transductive Logic*

Transductive Logic entails believing that an event closely preceding another in time, regardless of relationship, causes the second event. An erroneous causal link exists here. And since all causal links are erroneous, this really confuses people. Maybe you wonder how I can state that there are no causal links. I would suggest that when variables appear to exist in a causal relationship, we are actually viewing a correlational relationship. We find a temporal link but not cause. All variables over time contribute to the eventual "Cause". Someone who combines egocentricity with transductive logic believes they cause other people's behavior and that their behavior is about them. This constitutes part of the dynamic that keeps people in abusive relationships. Through inductive logic an abused person may ironically come to believe they are "bad" because the other person is misbehaving! This dynamic becomes a powerful influence in shaping the beliefs of abused children that then carry over into adulthood.

Here's an example of a statement driven by transductive logic. "Every time I care about someone they leave me." You might start by loosening the logic a little by asking:

> So do those people you don't care about stay with you, and have *you* ever *left* anybody who *cares* about *you*? But you think that your care causes people to leave you and this tempts you to abandon your care, leaving you feeling a void, which is a feeling you really want to avoid leaving your care—because caring never made any-one leave. And if you could really cause people to leave, then you

could also cause people to stay, now couldn't you? So this only proves that you neither cause people to leave nor stay, so your care is not guilty and you can keep your care and leave your worry to feel more care [the wording is so that the state of worry can receive the benefits and modify when connecting with the state of care] not worrying about caring. And what made you think you needed to protect your care in the first place by hiding it away? Why not let your care take care of you? Regularly fill yourself with care and then extend this outward to others. It's just sharing, with no obligation, you know? And now how do you feel about your caring, knowing it does not make people leave?

You can work toward a more constructive outcome from here.

Theme: Identify what the client believes to be the cause of their problem.

Questions to ask:

1. What does the client believe set this problem in motion? There was a time before the problem, then event X occurred, and the supposed problem was born. You want to elicit an answer that gives a timeline of events from which it emerges when the started.
2. Combining egocentricity with transductive logic, what appears to be the specific source within the self that triggered the problem—something like a limiting belief or resource-limiting state?

You may also find that the client engages in unspoken or spoken transductive logic that blocks *future* action. They may think or believe that certain behavior will have bad consequences. This also displays egocentricity because this person believes themself or their behavior to be the cause of evil outcomes in the past *and* future. Talk about a double bind!

VII. Animism

Animism attributes living qualities, thoughts, or emotions to inanimate objects. From English classes you may remember this concept as *personification* and the process as *personifying*. Personification is not necessarily dangerous and can be quite fun. The walls have ears, the sky is angry, and those brownies are calling to me—just a few examples. Sometimes attributing animate qualities to states of mind or beliefs appears to bring a state of mind or belief to life; it may then seem to direct itself independently of the individual's control.

A benefit of animistic thought is that it can offer a point of entry for hypnotic language into the listener's logic. By conferring living qualities on an inanimate objects, you may not only communicate with someone at the cognitive level of the problem, but you may also bypass a power struggle by attributing therapeutic ideas or suggestions to a third party. This third party source of suggestions can keep the therapist out of the authority figure role.

Animism may include the *meant to bes* of a belief system. Animism here means that the person attributes living, self-directing qualities to states, beliefs, and the environment or world. This superstitious mind set may also take a pessimistic form.

Sometimes animism may show up within the supposed cause of the problem, coming across as rather paranoid. The animistic process may resemble transductive logic. If I adopt behavior X, something bad will happen. Does behavior X solely cause the problem to occur (transductive), or does the environment seem to take it upon itself to strike back (animism)? Animism may also take the form of a symbol representing an unconscious part—the eagle within me, for example.

Sometimes you can inject animism into a rather self-limiting statement made by a client. Notice that injecting animism may allow for more comfortable discussion, as the individual's emotions are now dissociated from self and attributed to an item that possesses neither rational nor emotional capacity. For example, your client says, "There is no end in sight." You might respond by saying:

> I wonder how your eyes feel about their sight being limited. Do they feel guilty or frustrated, or maybe they just don't know that they have a limited view, so they can stop feeling bad about what they do not yet see, knowing they will see more compared to what they see now. It is not their fault that they cannot see beyond their range of vision.

But your eyes thought that what they saw was everything, or that they were supposed to be able to see everything; they believed their limited sight was all there was to see. I now wonder, and you may wonder too, what your eyes feel, realizing that there is much they cannot see, just like looking up at the sky on a clear night and thinking the stars you see are the only stars and you can see the whole of the universe, but you know *better*, don't you? And you can bet, that each eye knows more now, so that your mind can tell your eyes and your eyes can tell your mind that each appreciates the other and what they can see, remembering also to appreciate what you cannot see but know is there as well. Isn't that comforting now?

Theme: Identify the animate qualities attributed to inanimate objects such as states, beliefs, behaviors, objects in the environment, or the relationship with the universe—for example, "Life is out to get me!"

Question to ask:

1. Some form of illogic is likely present in an individual's states, beliefs, or behaviors. What animate qualities are attributed to inanimate objects or concepts? For example, a female client who goes over to her extremely dysfunctional mother's house says, "Every time I go over there, it's like the house makes bad things happen: it's got bad vibes. I always end up crying by the time I leave."

Notice how each of these cognitive categories interacts with the other. Rarely, if ever, does someone just use one of these styles to create a problem. If you use one, you almost certainly draw on two or three, or all, of these cognitive styles. They combine to form a cognitive gestalt that is usually limiting in terms of awareness, emotions, and behavioral choices. If you remove one part of the gestalt, one cognitive style, punching a hole in the boat, it will sink the whole gestalt, enabling you to replace it with a more seaworthy craft.

Beliefs and Emotional States

In this brief section, we will explore the role of beliefs and emotional states, the fourth tier, in processing information. This is included at the end of the chapter about cognitive styles since the discussion on beliefs-states is minimal and logically ends the discussion of this topic. The dynamics of beliefs and emotional states contain hidden powers that can make a significant difference in life choices. Very often our emotional states and beliefs result from the amount of information we take into consideration, how we perceive this, and the type of cognitive processing to which the information is subjected. We may not really consider that we possess choice when it comes to emotional states and beliefs. We may often just react to situations rather than be proactive in influencing the situations we face. It is being proactive that grants us opportunities for significant personal change.

The two elements making up the fourth tier, emotional states and beliefs, operate in concert whenever possible. There is a drive for congruity between these two elements. Cognitive dissonance (Festinger, 1957) describes the drive to align beliefs with behavior. We may also use cognitive dissonance to describe the discrepancy between emotional states and beliefs and the resulting drive to align the two. If we notice a discrepancy between how we feel emotionally and what we believe about self, life, or others, we experience an uneasy feeling of cognitive dissonance.

To illustrate cognitive dissonance, I'll use the example of a person who deflects compliments she receives from other people. Consider a woman who believes that others don't like her. As therapists, we know that it is really *she* who does not like herself. But as this woman makes her way through life, she believes that others do not like her. In spite of her perhaps avoiding others, she still encounters a person every now and then who pays her a compliment. But receiving and believing such compliments leads to a feeling of discomfort within her.

To accept the compliment would jeopardize her beliefs about herself and others, forcing her to change her emotional stance toward herself from general dislike to one of actually liking herself. Therefore, she must reject the compliment to reduce the sense of imbalance and uneasy feeling, thus maintaining congruency between her belief and her emotional state. However, if sufficient strength can be injected into a new, positive view of herself, this woman will change her emotional state to correspond with a positive belief self-evaluation.

Personal change can also come about just as effectively by changing the emotional state first. Beliefs about self, life, and others will then change in a like manner. In shifting to a resourceful, positive emotional state, one's beliefs about oneself change for the better. Since beliefs and emotional states need to reflect each other, we find that the fourth tier can exert a strong influence on an individual's functioning ability.

A certain interaction takes place between the fourth tier and the three tiers below. Accessing and functioning from the fourth tier can result from the processing of information that happens in the lower three tiers, a reactive state-belief. However, a *proactive* state may also be brought about by the emotional state and beliefs held at the fourth tier. If we choose our emotional state and our beliefs, we naturally create a corresponding alignment in our cognitive processing, perception, and awareness.

Examining emotional states-beliefs in action in everyday life, we observe that self-defeating behaviors and successful recoveries exemplify corrective action to restore state-belief congruence. You can intervene with a client by changing a state to alter beliefs. Or you can intervene by changing beliefs to alter and ameliorate an emotional state. If you successfully change either the belief or the state, the other dimension will naturally follow, aligning itself.

One of the most potent opportunities for personal change comes from choosing what we will believe about self, life, or others or from what emotional state we will live our lives. Once we choose a belief or a state and live from this position, further choices align with this chosen belief or state. The consequences may profoundly alter our lives.

The dynamics of the four tiers mean that each exerts an influence on the other three. The highest tier, emotions-beliefs, may exert the most influence on the whole system of information processing. But changing any one of the four may lead to changes in the other three. This is the reason that this book consists of four categories of hypnotic language interventions. Changing one does not always change the other three. But if change is carefully made in one of the four tiers, this change will have an inevitable ripple effect, creating a new balance among the four tiers.

I have categorized the hypnotic language patterns in subsequent chapters to reflect points of entry into this four-tier information-processing system. The four categories of hypnotic language that I use in this work include *emotional states, perception, time orientation, and behavior.* Each of these categories of hypnotic language represents ways of influencing our awareness, gestalt-making, cognitive processes, and emotional states-beliefs. Changing emotional states to create personal change has already been discussed. Initiating personal change through altering perception has likewise been discussed.

There is good reason for using behavioral change to result in personality change. Different behavior creates a new set of consequences in life. This new set of consequences resulting from different behavior permits different life experiences, new awareness, new perception, new cognitive processing, and new emotional states-beliefs. The former gestalt of the four-tier information-processing system becomes disarranged, creating dissonance and possibilities for change in life.

This leaves changing behavior and altering time orientation as two other avenues of personal change yet to be explained. Changing time orientation represents an interesting, perhaps more subtle, influence in bringing about personal change. There are several elements that combine to encapsulate life experience, conferring on it existence as a separate memory. Time is one of the elements that bind an experience together into a memory, for memory is time-dependent. Two questions asked when reviewing a past event are "when did it happen?" and "for how long did it happen?" If we access the time-dependent organization of memory, we gain an opportunity to open the memory, then to access the four tiers of information processing to initiate change.

The following chapters will present a variety of hypnotic language scripts. The four categories (emotional states, perception, time orientation, and behavior) that these scripts represent offer potent points of entry into understanding and intervening in the dynamics of personal problems. While you may find that the language patterns presented here possess some traits similar to other categories, I have organized them by their primary theme used in addressing client issues. Each of the four categories begins by presenting a case study. This includes client dynamics and resulting dysfunction. I then explain the reasoning behind the hypnotic language chosen for intervention. Following these case examples, numerous hypnotic language patterns are presented that target specific issues utilizing the four categories. I'll explain each language pattern before it is presented.

Chapter 4
Hypnotic Language Scripts Addressing Emotional States

This chapter focuses on the use of hypnotic language to address and change emotional states. A case example illustrates the influence of emotional states in creating personal problems and their symptoms. This case description and transcript, also illustrate the use of hypnotic language in changing emotional states, thereby offering solutions to problems. Numerous examples of hypnotic language addressing emotional states follow this case presentation, each preceded by the rationale behind the hypnotic language pattern.

Treating Irritable Bowel Syndrome

We begin with a case example of using hypnotic language to treat irritable bowel syndrome. This case is included in this chapter, as irritable bowel syndrome may be thought of as arising from an uncomfortable and tension-producing state of emotion. The hypnotic script in this case is one that I used in treating, Adam, a 12-year-old boy. He had experienced more than two years of intractable stomach pain without any detectable organic source. The pain was reportedly present during most of this period. He missed so many days of school that he had to be home-schooled in order to keep up and pass his grades. The stomach pain disrupted his sleep and appetite, as well as restricted his lifestyle outside of school. His pain incapacitated him at times. Adam had been examined and evaluated by numerous physicians and treated with many different medications to no avail.

Adam came in for his initial evaluation and all subsequent sessions accompanied by his mother. He presented as a very intelligent, well-behaved boy with a variety of interests in life. However, due to his condition he had not been able to pursue these interests for more than two years. Some depression was evident. His mother Alice evidenced considerable anxiety and frustration about his condition. During the course of Adam's initial evaluation, we explored his interests, likes, and dislikes, as well as his goals for the near- and long-term future.

One of the primary pieces of information that I wanted to identify was when, where, and how Adam felt most relaxed, happy, and satisfied. Adam told me that he especially enjoyed going to a small piece of property owned by his family outside his hometown. The family owned a small cabin adjacent to a lake. The lake is a private one and a place where Adam found great peace. He would often follow the short path from the cabin to the lake, either with family or on his own. Sometimes he would put on a life jacket, get in the dinghy, and row across the lake. Adam told me that handling the boat by himself was a very recent accomplishment permitted by his mother and father. He displayed great pride in this accomplishment.

Realizing that being in the boat on the lake was one of Adam's favorite experiences and that beneficial resource states were associated with it, I decided to generate a script around his being on the lake in the boat. Also, this recent advance of Adam's "going solo" in the boat represented a positive developmental step toward increasing personal independence and becoming more self-directed. Some of this boy's distress may have revolved around negotiating developmental steps, as he and his mother appeared to be rather over-aligned, while his father, by report, appeared somewhat distant.

Adam may have been wrestling, in part, with transitional family dynamics brought on by his growing up. He was moving ever closer to independence and to eventually leaving home. Being an only child, his leaving home would then place his parents face to face with each other in what may have become a somewhat emotionally distant marriage. Armed with this information about the family dynamics, Adam's symptoms, and restrictions on his lifestyle, we set out to help him find and recover necessary resources that would enable him to function better in a variety of settings.

During the remainder of the first session, I laid the groundwork for future sessions. I developed a simple induction drawing on his positive feelings about the lake he and his family visited; I wanted to provide an initial opportunity for Adam to learn how to relax. As I talked, describing the lake scene and drawing on multiple senses, he seemed to relax significantly. But, in about five to seven minutes, he pulled himself out of the trance state, to say the process felt good. I explained how this good feeling would become even better and last longer when he continued relaxing while I evoked the pleasant lake setting.

At this point, I was concerned that he might be bidding for control by coming out of trance on his own. In the hope of bypassing this struggle (if this was happening), I told him that I trusted him and his ability to relax. I told him that I was convinced that since he knew what to do to relax, he could practice this on his own at home, relaxed and stay relaxing even more deeply and staying relaxed for longer. I told Adam that he should practice this deep relaxation just as much as he wanted to feel better. We seemed to maintain a positive rapport and I set an appointment for the near future.

In the next session, Adam seemed generally upbeat and said he had practiced relaxing and did feel somewhat better when he practiced. But he had also suffered some significant stomach pains outside of his practice times. We agreed that in this session, I would talk to him for an extended time, while he would just listen until I told him we were finished.

We agreed to my talking to him and his listening all the way through as we began the formal process of hypnotherapy, Adam preferred to lie on the floor with a thick area rug as his mattress. Once he arranged himself comfortably, I presented the following metaphorical narrative:

> Since you've been down to your parents' cabin and the nearby lake many times, Adam, I'm sure this is very familiar to you. I imagine you may have a particular path you walk on as you go to the lake, so you can begin imagining this now. You go out the front door and begin walking. As you walk, you may hear and feel a crunching from the path beneath your feet.

With each step you take, moving you closer to the lake, you can feel the ground under your feet. This familiar path that you've taken to the lake so many times has a sort of slant to it as you slowly making your way closer and closer to the lake. Maybe you begin thinking about how it will look when you see it again. Maybe you begin to feel that certain feeling of calm and comfort and joy that you get there, now.

Once the lake comes into sight, you may take a minute or so to just sort of scan the lake. Maybe you notice the shoreline. You may notice how the water looks as it just touches up against the moist soil. And you can notice how the shoreline changes as you take a look all along the shore. Maybe at some points it sort of curved. And maybe at some other points it's almost straight. And as you take a look along the whole line of the lake shore, you notice just how big the lake is and notice how the water color changes just a bit as the water is further from the shore and deeper.

Once you've looked around the whole lake, you decide to walk over to the dock. You notice the wooden boards and how they look. Now, stepping up on the boards, you observe how they feel…and maybe there's a certain sound each time you step on the boards. You decide to walk over to the small boat tied there to the dock. Stepping carefully into the boat, you sit down gently. Untying the boat from the dock, you push off, noticing how you start to glide across the water. Observe how you start rowing quickly, then slow down, but you slow very slowly and now are just drifting calmly. And as you drift, there is silence. You floating on top of the water in this drifting boat, totally quiet, absorbed in the sights, smells, and feel of the lake.

As you drift slowly, gently across the water, you notice some gentle ripples that spread out from the boat. Maybe you notice just one and follow it as it slides across the surface of the water. It may be that it starts out quickly, with a bit of a wave. But as it moves further and further away from the boat, it gets smaller and smaller, sort of fading away. And maybe you decide to watch just a particular spot on the water, watching each ripple pass through this spot. And as each ripple passes, you find that you become this much more relaxed, more and more relaxed. As you count the ripples from 1 to 10 you find you become the most relaxed. I'll count them for you so you can just watch and feel…more and more relaxed.

One, feeling calm and relaxed, gently floating….Two, noticing that you notice an even deeper calm; and this relaxed feeling becomes this much more pleasant….Three, feeling it through your whole self....Four, as you notice these gentle ripples gliding by, all the while you become more and more relaxed, just floating....Five, noticing how you find this feeling of calm relaxation increasingly deeper and more pleasant as you sit floating in the boat floating on the water, supported so well and safely....Six, the next ripple brings you this much more deeply into this feeling of the most relaxed you can imagine....Just drifting, noticing how you ever so gently sway a bit back and forth, back and forth as you glide so slowly on the water. Seven, this much more relaxed as you find you feel a comfortable and comforting feeling....Eight, continuing to feel an even greater sense of calm...enjoying this more and more as you feel this more and more to your liking....Nine, so very relaxed, so deeply relaxed and....Ten, deeper still.

And as you gently float and drift on the water, you may decide to use one oar and just move yourself toward a part of the lake that looks interesting. Maybe you've seen this part before, but someway it looks different now. Maybe you notice something you had not noticed before. Maybe it's the way the water meets the shoreline or maybe it's the shape of the land over there. But either way, you make your way gradually over there, slowly drifting up to the shore. Once there you move the boat up to and on the shore so you can step out and on the wet ground. You get your footing and decide to walk up the shore, investigating the bushes and flowers there. You may notice some trees and maybe you walk to where the trees start but you still notice the sunlight. And as you look around you look down at the ground and you notice something shining up at you.

You notice this interesting, shiny stone on the ground. Bending down to pick it up you find how amazingly light this is. It feels as though it must be hollow. It is so light it barely feels like you have anything in your hand. You look at it and notice the color variations. You see some shades of gray, lighter and darker. You see some shades of brown and gold and even some near-white colors. It looks so interesting that you decide to just slowly, lightly slide your fingertip across the surface. How incredibly smooth it feels. You lightly glide your fingertip across again and it is so smooth that it feels like it was polished. It's odd even. And you just continue feeling the lightness and the smoothness. It feels so interesting that you just continue touching it and noticing the smoothness.

This stone is so unusual that you decide to take it with you. You put it in your pocket and it is amazing, so light that it feels like there is nothing there. Yet you know it is and how smooth it is, smooth and light. You sometimes just touch your pocket just to remember how light and smooth. With this interesting and appealing stone in your pocket you make your way back to the boat. You step in and once again gently push off to go back across the water. All the while you notice and remember this incredibly smooth, light stone and how it feels, so smooth.

Slowly you glide across the water and reach the middle of the lake. And finally you return to the dock. You secure the boat and step out on to the wooden dock remembering this most interesting, smooth, light item you carry with you. You can't even feel it in your pocket but you know it's there. You start back on the familiar path that leads from the lake back to the cabin. And with each step you gradually start to become more and more aware of the place you are in now. And I'll count those steps for you.

Ten, gradually making your way along the path that leads you back home. Nine, all the while you walk you notice and remember the smooth, light stone and how it looks and feels. Each step leads you closer to home…Eight, as you carry with you this most interesting and appealing stone. The path looks familiar and yet it somehow feels different because you know you have with you this most interesting stone of such lightness that it barely feels present, and yet you know it is. Seven, moving this much closer to home. Six, all the while you carry in the back of your mind the knowledge that you carry with you this light, smooth most appealing feeling. Five and Four…you to benefit remember, feeling this presence of this comfortable and comforting light, smooth feeling. Three, nearly returning home all the while different everywhere you go, no matter where. You remember in the back of your mind and remember and feel this smooth, flat, light feeling that feels so good. Two, noticing the places you go, some familiar and some different and new, this feeling continues with you because you carry this reminder everywhere you go. One, gradually returning here in this room, remembering and feeling what you now know and feel everywhere.

As he begins to stir, I say, "There you go, just right. You can take your time waking up here. How do you feel?" Adam stated that he felt fine. He reported being pain free. We talked a bit more and processed his trance experience. He remained in the office with his mother a few more minutes as we talked. We decided to reschedule once more in a few weeks to assess his status and do additional intervention if needed. At this next session, Adam reported that he had been pain free since our last visit. We decided that treatment was complete for now. We discussed the benefits gained and the old opportunities regained as well as new opportunities now available for Adam to enjoy.

Several months after the last contact, his mother called to schedule another appointment. Adam had been pain-free for several months when his stomach pain recurred to a mild degree. When he came in for our session, Adam described intermittent stomach pains in the last couple of weeks. We took a return visit to the lake scene. By the time we finished the hypnosis and he came out of trance, Adam was again pain-free. It has been over nine months without any contact from Adam's mother, which I take to mean that Adam continues living without pain.

Walking in Comfort: Reducing Anxiety

The treatment pattern described next is designed to help shift a person from an anxiety reaction in a particular situation to a relaxed, calm response to the same situation. The particular content includes childhood settings. If the client's childhood was traumatic, this treatment pattern should not to be offered. The use of wine is included, so first determine your client's feelings about wine because some clients' have adverse feelings about wine and its use. Please be sure to take into account your client's past and values. Assist the client into a light-to-moderate depth trance. Then present the following language to help transport the client from anxiety to comfort about a particular situation.

> As you find this deep state of relaxation and calm, so magnetic that you just focus on it completely, consider a time, and maybe you've experienced this or maybe you can just imagine a time when you re-visited the home you grew up in. Maybe you drove there and as you got closer and closer to the house you noticed familiar land-marks and thought back to pleasant experiences you had there when you were young. And when you get to your old house, you notice what had seemed like a huge yard…now seems very small. And what had seemed like a huge house…now seems very small. Interesting how, as your grow up, things from you past become smaller.

You may go inside the house, in your mind, and notice what was your room and what was your closet. And maybe you can think about and notice what had been your clothes and maybe your shoes. You can notice how these clothes and shoes no longer fit you as you have grown and are bigger than this now. And you can think about all the things from the past that you've outgrown because… you have.

And while your old shoes may have at one time been a size 5 or 6, these are just numbers now and though numbers are never wrong, just sometimes they are sometimes wrong when used at the wrong times. And time uses numbers in a particular sequence, so that it will always be 3 o'clock after 2 o'clock and it will always be 11 o'clock after 10 o'clock. And maybe you've had the experience when you knew the night before you wanted to get up in the morning at a particular time and so you set the alarm, just to be sure, but your unconscious mind already knew and woke you just before, so you did not need the alarm.

And time marches on and you know that you can set your own internal clock so that you can stop the alarm and, instead…deeply relax at just the right time., and you know just when, so that you can march on in time and notice curiously notice how when your feet touch the…grow more and more calm, relaxed, and wonderfully pleased.

And this interesting, pleasant feeling, you can savor like a fine meal, appreciating each morsel and even before, noticing the presentation and the scent, causing you to sink into a deeper, more relaxed state, during each piece you fully appreciate as much as you desire the sampling of each item, which you fully appreciate to the depth of your being, and after the meal also savoring like the right choice of wine finds and satisfies the spot.

Sometimes we get an itch for something special and you know that only this will satisfy this itch that you scratch, feeling the relief gradually and then fully all the way through, basking in this relief and relaxing.

And sometimes one itches enough.

So that you can, you know, use what you know to satisfy what you know…you need…you will from this point forward finding great delight in each opportunity to do this each time you do. And I don't know when, but you will just remember these most pleasant feelings and notice within as you feel and naturally express this feeling and be able to re-create them within yourself, whether it will be the very idea of going to a particular place when you first and most feel these feelings, or it will be on the way to some location as you notice the location of these exceptionally pleasant feelings within, or maybe you will feel the most when you arrive and go inside to find and feel the presence in the present, enjoying this sort of secret within as you go within. And then again, you may find that you find you feel these best of feelings all the while you are there and hear this within yourself, remembering and feeling on and on, stretching well into your future and the comforting reassurance this brings you.

The Bee Sting and the Antihistamine: Stress Response

The hypnotic language pattern that follows is designed for someone who tends to overreact to minor stress or challenges. The intent of the story is to convey both the temporary nature of distress and an alternative response to the usual overreaction. Those who overreact often expect the worst and activate their response so quickly that often they have not fully assessed a given situation.

This script was used in treating a woman who tended to overreact to daily challenges in her workplace. This client was an office manager within a multi-physician medical practice. Her job placed her squarely between the staff interacting with patients and the administrative staff. Her mid-level management role meant that she was under pressure from each side of the company—from the employees she managed and those who managed her. At times she felt caught in the middle between these two forces. To some extent she felt helpless, yet charged with overseeing day-to-day operations and ensuring they went smoothly.

Barbara would experience stress from either or both these two sides at work, the managed or the managing. In response to this stress, Barbara would consistently respond in a way that effectively assessed the problem and then would devise a reasonable solution. But, in the process of problem solving, she would develop two primary problems. One is that she would eat unhealthy foods to ease her stress. The other stress response she experienced was breaking out in a red rash across her neck and upper chest.

Barbara came to me for relief from what she knew was an unnecessary stress response that brought unwanted consequences. In the process of assessing the dynamics at her workplace, it was determined that she tended to think the worst would happen in response to any given problem. She tended to over-respond internally; she would activate an internal alarm and this, in turn, would activate her physiology, so that she got a skin rash and was overcome by a desire for food to calm herself. Even though Barbara always found effective solutions for the day-to-day challenges that came up while managing the medical practice, she tended to doubt her abilities and thus to react with more intensity than was necessary. This excessive intensity set in motion her symptoms.

The script below was aimed at addressing the problems that came to Barbara's attention and also to addressing her overreaction, its consequences, as well as present her with alternatives. This script also addresses Barbara's tendency to use potentially negative consequences as a motivator. The dynamics of the solution presented in the script plays to her existing motivational style rather than trying to shift the basis of her motivation. Barbara responded very well to this brief intervention. Follow-up six months later revealed that she had not experienced any further rashes and that she had lost weight by not engaging in stress eating.

> This is a story about a woman who was outside...playing, or was she working? Well, either way, she was outside and things seemed to be going well when all of a sudden a bee stung her. She naturally grabbed the area that hurt, where she had been stung, and noticed a red spot that had begun to swell. She became concerned and began to wonder how much this was going to hurt and how the redness and swelling going would increase. She'd heard of people who had such a bad reaction to bee stings that they got very sick and some even died.
>
> So this woman raced inside...and immediately found medicine that was made to control allergic reactions. Without thinking, she took two of these pills and hoped for the best. Scared and worried, she

watched the sting site with great interest. Within just a few minutes she began to sort of…lose focus on the sting as the intensity began…decreasing. She noticed the pain was much less and the stinging was nearly gone… having done nothing but observe. All this happened in just a few minutes. The redness was fading; instead of a solid bright redness, it was now fading and becoming splotchy to even less. Her reaction…had passed. This relief took just a few minutes and the two pills she'd *gulped* down had yet to even take effect. Now she'd have to endure the enduring effects of these two pills for four hours to come. If she'd only known or trusted…her body naturally knows…how to stop reacting and simply overlook such minor stings and just move on…she could be well over…and done with the injury without adding any insult to it. Well, lesson learned.

So she now knows that with many injuries, relief is just a few minutes away. And further, you don't have to hurt yourself to know you can heal. Now she knows and anticipates…even anticipates anticipating…experiencing relief immediately, *now*.

So soon…she feels relief, smiling, as she knows…All the times and places she will know and experience this with great delight like a secret she keeps inside that protects and comforts…Always present.

Baby Tooth: Maturing

This metaphor addresses limiting beliefs that we may form during childhood. These beliefs stem from the very limited cognitive abilities that we possess during our childhood. Very often, as we develop more advanced and complex thinking abilities with age, we modify childhood beliefs. But we often forget to update some of our earliest and most potent beliefs. Sometimes the beliefs formed during childhood in the midst of a trauma are the ones we revert to and do not update. These early traumas seem to become encapsulated, even neurologically, shut off from updates since the event.

Perhaps we don't update these traumatically motivated beliefs because they seem so powerful and emotion laden that we try to ignore them in order to feel more comfortable. Maybe we ignore these childhood beliefs because they seemed life-saving at the time and we don't want to risk the consequences of tinkering with such important material. And maybe these beliefs formed through trauma exist in a sort of cognitive vacuum, severed from the rest of our growing knowledge and cognitive abilities. Thus, we don't even consciously realize that we need to update. Regardless, these unexamined beliefs exert considerable influence on our lives, and what once felt life-preserving may later become life-limiting.

The language pattern below starts of with utilizing confusion through time disorientation and an inverse correlation. Why, this explanation is confusing in itself! The purpose below is to help dissociate the client from whatever current clutch they may have on some unresolved issue. The overall process of the pattern offers a transition from early childhood through adulthood, noticing developmental landmarks along the way that remind us of increased capacity and more advanced abilities for dealing with and resolving issues as we mature.

> It is interesting to note that our old beliefs are from our youth and our young beliefs are from our older age. Sometimes in life, no matter when, everyone's had the experience of finding that some things do not fit. Maybe we are an adult and we try on some shoes and find they are either too big for our feet or too small. Maybe we try on some pants and find they are too big for us or we're too big. And sometimes a dog pants. And sometimes a dog barks up the wrong tree. Maybe this mistake, in search for something important, can be corrected.

> When a child is born, and when you were, he develops teeth at just the right time so he can eat solid food that provides good nutrition, and different nourishment than what he first needed. Surely teeth develop in coordination with the stomach's advancing ability to digest more substantial food. And, in turn, this solid food also provides an opportunity for more advanced functioning in the stomach and intestines. This more complex food also contributes to further development and growth of the child into an adult.

> These first teeth that a child gets are sometimes known as baby teeth or temporary teeth. These teeth are just right for the task at hand. But these teeth are a sort of a practice set, a warm up set if you will, to be replaced later by what's known as permanent teeth. During childhood, teeth begin developing out of site, in the gums. As these teeth develop, they grow bigger and begin to put some

pressure on the temporary teeth as they push through to the surface. The stronger, more substantial teeth, designed for a life-time, begin to dislodge the baby teeth, loosening them one at a time.

It's about the same time you learn...to write that...this...happens.

And you can imagine how at first the child and the baby teeth them-selves might begin to worry about this chain of events. My gosh! I'm loosing my teeth and I just barely got used to having them and they were so useful, what now? And the teeth must feel quite anxious as they notice and feel their security slipping away. But the looser these baby teeth get the less useful they are. The baby teeth get looser and looser, developing a wobble now that tempts one to wiggle the tooth back and forth.

Behind the scenes, nature is at work. It almost seems instinctive to play with and wiggle this ever-loosening tooth. We may think this tooth play is by choice but maybe it's just a natural progression designed to let the old give way to the better suited new. At some deeper level, part of you knows this baby tooth has to leave. These baby teeth were never meant to last. They were never designed to stay. Rather, these teeth were designed to be released, never kept, so that more advanced, more able teeth can take their place and do a better job. This natural way also gets rewarded by what happens afterward. Everyone remembers the tooth fairy experience. It's very interesting how nature and society conspire to help one release and replace old outdated items with those that fit and function better and provide more opportunities with greater ease as you look from here noticing the many and new opportunities and ways that you can sink your teeth into life.

Encased in Ice: Recovering from Childhood Abuse

This metaphor addresses issues surrounding childhood abuse. The story's principal point is that our inner self, our healthy, natural self, can remain safe and untouched from abuse in spite of external assault. Before telling this story, it is important to establish a state of safety and comfort so the listener will be optimally receptive. Conflict and resolution within the story are presented while inten-tionally invoking worried anticipation about the future status of precious items (such as the buds and eventual fruit of citrus trees). The metaphor is intended to convey how we can find ways of naturally protecting our inner self, enabling us to endure trauma. We can then release this protective coating or shell when conditions are safe, allowing the self to bloom and be fruitful.

Also notice how the verb tense changes throughout the story. The early part, invoking present safety, is in the present tense. The portion containing the unresolved conflict is in the past tense, dissociating the listener from the trauma by placing it in the past. The outcome or future is told in both present and future tense. This tense shifting is done to set the trauma in the past, separating the listener from it. The resolution and consequences of this resolved trauma are presented in present and future verb form for more effective orientation in time and accessing of healthy resources.

> This is an interesting story that a friend of my cousin told me. Now since this story is at least once, if not twice, removed, you can decide if it's true for yourself. My cousin's friend used to live in Florida when she was younger. She lived in the part of the country where farmers grow citrus fruit. You know, grapefruits, oranges, and other citrus fruits. She enjoyed being down there and she especially enjoyed the beach and the great fun she had there.
>
> One year this girl and her friend decided they would take a trip to the beach. She and her friend wanted to choose just the right time to go to the beach. You know, when the water would be warm enough to swim in comfortably. Not like some of the cold snaps that happen down there that make the water so bitter and endanger the growing citrus fruits. And so this girl and her friend head to the beach and, sure enough, the water is very warm, much like bath water. You know how you can draw a bath and how a bath can draw you in, feeling the relaxing comfort. You sort of become one with the warm water and the comfort, and it becomes you.
>
> This girl really appreciated the warmth of the current and she also remembered, from her comfortable warm spot in the water, the past spring, and how cold it had been. She remembered how much different the water temperature was then, although it was warm now. And she remembered how the fruit growers worried about their groves of fruit trees as the unexpected cold weather descended and lasted into the spring. It was a time of great uncertainty. But she also remembered the amazing solution that saved the fruits.

I want to tell you this story of how the fruit growers discovered to their surprise how they could save their crops. So maybe this story won't be new to you but while you listen you may discover some things that you have…yet…knew at a deeper level.

Sometimes, even in the spring the air gets very cold there in Florida and the temperature can go below freezing. This threatens to freeze the buds on the citrus trees, which will stop their development. And this one spring the farmers discovered an ingenious method for keeping the vulnerable, fragile new buds safe. Maybe it first happened without really planning it but it worked when they noticed what happened afterwards. And it's what happens afterwards that matters the most.

When the weather gets really cold in Florida and the temperature is supposed to go below freezing, threatening the citrus tree buds, the growers actually leave their water sprinkler systems on overnight. And, as I said, the first time this happened it may have been unplanned, after they saw what happened the farmers used this method again and again.

These sprinkler systems are very advanced and run very deep. Normally they can sense when to come on and when to go off each day and night, which is very important because it may be easy to know when to start something, but how do you know when to stop? These sprinkler systems somehow know how to sense that the old condition, absence of moisture, is no longer. And once they sense this, they stop, because too much is as bad as not enough.

The growers, on this particularly cold night, kept the sprinklers on all night until just after dawn. Now at first they were not sure what was going to happen. And so much was riding on this, their very future. So they worried and fretted, sleeping little and wondering a lot about what would happen.

What *did* happen is that the water from the sprinklers that covered the buds gradually got colder and colder as the air cooled. Eventually the water froze on the buds, and the more water that accumulated on the buds, the more layers of ice formed. At first the growers thought that this would surely harm the fruit buds, dooming them for sure. But what actually happened surprised them. It turned out that the ice that formed on the buds was just barely below freezing. These citrus buds can handle temperatures just below freezing, and so the ice provided a protective coating that kept the buds from getting any colder, even though the air temperature got colder.

Interestingly, the layers of ice saved the buds from a true hard freeze that *would* have permanently damaged them.

Well, the growers did not know this yet, and so they got up very early the next morning to find out the results of this experiment. They watched the sprinklers continue watering, coating the citrus buds. Once the night was over and gave way to dawn, the sprinklers stopped and the temperature rose. Now, the warming air gradually softens the hard ice, melting away the layers from the outside inward as the sun radiates its warmth. The buds on the trees become more and more visible as their delicate colors and textures can be seen in more detail, having come through the danger to now more fully emerge as the conditions are safe and more than this really, growth producing and supporting.

Now, the weather encourages the bud to grow. The warmth received, signals the bud to continue developing, emerging to receive this much more warmth and sunlight that continues the growing process, breaking through, not just the ice that melted and evaporated but also the protective shell of the bud is now gradually becoming a thing of the past, no longer needed as the bud grows able to flourish as the conditions are right, outgrowing its former protective shell. The bud, now flowering, knows exactly how to do this from the inside out, becoming…itself.

This woman immersed in warm water continues appreciating and enjoying the water's warmth, noticing how much has changed and how much more she can do as a result of current conditions. She can just bask in the sun and feel its warmth, she can stroll along the beach, noticing how moving forward brings a change in scenery; she can swim, float, or play in the waves. She is able to choose what she likes and enjoys most according to her taste at the time, knowing what to look for and what to avoid. During these days and those that follow, this woman continues to remember ways of enjoying safe fun. From this point forward she knows how to use her knowledge and experiences in the present to create the future she wants.

In a different way, knowing safety, degrees and amounts to the right way.

And you can gradually or more quickly begin noticing the opportunities to choose in such a way that you choose what appeals to you and your deepest desires, allowing you to pursue and reach your goals, knowing the paths to choose, realizing, trusting your deepest healthiest awareness, trusting your intuition and instincts to lead you the right way, enjoying with great enthusiasm and eagerness, embracing the many opportunities now and in the future creating what you most desire and maintaining this.

Hose Kink: Recovering from Past Wounds

This metaphor addresses releasing and healing a past wound in order to develop new personal growth in the future. The story involves a vegetable garden and using a garden hose to bring life-sustaining water to the vegetables. In the process of trying to get the hose to reach the vegetables, the gardener finds the hose is stuck on something behind her, limiting the range of the watering hose (referencing a past wound that limits future growth). The story proceeds to describe ways the gardener tries to resolve the stuck spot. The resolution reveals how she does finally free herself in order to generate a free flow of water enabling new growth in the future.

This is a story about a gardener. This gardener has decided to make a vegetable garden at the back of her property. Jenny, we'll call her, looks out from the window at the back of her house and sees an opportunity. She sees where she can create something she's always wanted, a vegetable garden. So Jennie walks out to the back of her back yard to survey the area. She decides just how large an area of vegetables that part of the property will hold. She clears out the space nicely and amends the soil to make it this much more fertile and supportive to growing the vegetables of her choice. Jenny carefully selects the vegetables that she likes and the ones that her climate will support. Planning the plot and carefully planting, she places the seeds and plants in just the right order, positioning them according to their eventual size and needs for ultimate growing conditions.

The weather even cooperates in the early days and nights. Consistent, regular rain provides just the right growing conditions. Sunshine beamed in the days between rains so the garden was in great order for growing. Jenny would regularly walk out to the back of her back yard where the vegetables were planted and carefully take stock of each plant and seed as it grew. The weather continued to cooperate right through the early spring. Now real action was starting to take place as each day some noticeable growth was taking place. Her own enthusiasm was growing as well. She experienced such a sense of pride and accomplishment.

As the spring went along, the rain began decreasing and the amount and intensity of sunshine increased, drying the soil. Jenny kept careful tabs on the moisture in the soil so she would know just when to add water, maintaining the growth of these vegetables. She hoped for rain as the soil became drier and drier. She figured that sure as she was to water the garden there would come a heavy rain, making for too much moisture. She waited and waited but it became clear she would have to water the vegetables, even if it did rain.

So Jenny checked her watering hose and made sure it was well connected to the source, the faucet at the back of the house. She tightened it well and turned on the water. The plan was to just let the hose lay in the garden, moving it from time to time, soaking the ground well. Now she began pulling the hose, with the water pouring out of it, across the backyard. Further and further she walked along the yard deciding just where to water first. As Jenny walked quickly, not wanting to waste the water flowing out of the hose, she suddenly jerked to an abrupt halt, quite short of the garden. The water that was pouring out shrank to a trickle. Her first instinct was to pull hard on the hose. She did and found it actually hurt her arm as the hose would not give and now the water was just about choked off. Jenny looked from where she was down the line of the hose, tracing it back to the faucet. She noticed a sizable kink about two-thirds of the way back toward the faucet. She felt relief and frustration all at once. She went into a series of furious movements, twisting and rotating the end of the hose with her hand trying to unravel the kink. She twisted, turned, made sweeping up and down motions with her hand while holding the hose but to no avail. The hose would ripple all the way back to the kink but freeze there. Her frustration grew as all she wanted to do was water the vegetables and she did not want to walk all that distance back to where the kink was holding up progress. It seemed such a waste of time as she'd already gotten this far, just a few more feet would do it.

She paused for a moment and thought. The only way she was going to get this done was to just go ahead and go back to the kink and release it. This would take care of it once and for all. Jenny walked quickly with a purpose back to the kink and reached down, took the hose and turned it in such a way with several twists to straighten it out. It then laid flat and she looked at the far end of the hose and saw it jump anew with water gushing out of it. A smile of satisfaction came across Jenny's face as she'd made things right. She felt this within as well as she made her way back to the end of the hose, picked it up, and proceeded to place it carefully at just the right spot within the garden. She watched as the water flowed freely onto and into the soil as she imagined the moisture seeping deeper into the soil making its way to the roots, nourishing them and she thought about the growth this would produce combined with proper soil and sunshine… anticipating enjoying the harvest.

Mine Entrance: Accessing Resource States

The metaphor underlying this narrative addresses the conscious, unconscious, and potentially deeper levels of the unconscious. The language pattern is based on the idea that personal conflict stems from a battle for control between the conscious and unconscious mind. This includes the idea that there are certain emotional injuries that limit access to and expression of the unconscious mind. Such limiting emotional injuries and their debris enter the shallow depths of the unconscious mind through the conscious mind. These injuries then tend to interfere with retrieving the resources residing in our deeper, unconscious mind.

This story concerns a man who decides to go on a hike. When he hikes he likes to go with a friend. So he calls up his hiking buddy and they agree to go the next day. They choose their particular path and set off on the trail to discover what nature has in store for them along the way. While walking through the woods they enjoy the scenery, the trees, the plants and flowers, and a nearby stream. They notice the various wildlife and their instinctive activities, knowing just what to do, when and how. Then the men come upon what looks like a cave. From a distance, you know how sometimes things look one way until you get a closer look? It's sort of like when you see a scarecrow. From a distance it seems pretty menacing, but the closer you look, the less substantial it really is. As they take a closer look, approaching slowly, they can see an opening that leads into the cave. They are not sure how big or deep this cave is, but the closer they get the more they realize they can't yet see the end of it, which intrigues them and raises their curiosity.

Once they get up to the opening to the cave they see a bunch of debris that has accumulated around the mouth of the cave. There are some stones, several not too big but one that is quite large. There are also some tree branches that must have been blown off during a storm and landed in the opening. From a distance, they notice that there are sort of three layers, not lairs but layers. Outside the cave is a collection of things, some that have been there a long time and some that appear more recent, but all are exposed to the light. Then, near the mouth of the cave is a collection of debris that has accumulated from outside and landed just barely inside the cave. Beyond this, no debris exists and you can see clearly into the rest of the cave.

After sizing up the situation, they decide that they'll never really be able to tell how the debris got in the opening of the cave or where it came from. But they also decide that it's more important to remove the debris than knowing how it got there. Now, it took awhile to move all the clutter away from the cave. Each of them could move most of it on their own but to move some of the heavy pieces they had to work together since there were obstacles to move the out of the way.

Now, entering the cave, they see the light shining into the cave, illuminating the contents. And the deeper they go they find…the deeper they go…they find…more and more…treasures, years in the making…you go deeper…finding treasures centuries in the making…you go deeper, finding treasures centuries of centuries in the making…you aware. Finding…noticing…from all angles the different facets and the features, noticing the angles and how the light reflects showing you…what this can do, how and when the feeling this brings in you no matter what went in there it's what you bring out that valuable knowing this from the deepest depths are the rarest and most precious gems that have been in the making the longest time in the making them the most valuable and desirable. And you can search the depths of your riches, your filled inner self, and find what shines and what is most valuable and precious, bringing this out for the world to see and enjoy and benefiting all who experience it. After all, it is these riches that were made for you to bring out because this is where and how they do the most good. And this feeling the entire time you find, bring out and display, only enhancing with each step as you show the glow that illuminates. Noticing the many kinds, the many ways and the many, many more of these unique gems you possess and the more you bring out the more you bring out this wonderful feeling now and in your future, noticing the experiences you can have and will have leading to more…and…more.

Tee Shirts: Choosing States with Foresight

The hypnotic language below aims to utilize past learning and emotional states to increase foresight and awareness of choice for both present and future. The metaphor involves collecting tee shirts from various vacation locations and accessing the emotional states associated with each one. There is also an embedded metaphor addressing planning and foresight to enhance the selection of emotional states for present and future use. Several opportunities for additional embedded metaphors reside within this language pattern. The therapist could easily work with the baggage in the metaphor as emotional baggage and elaborate on the past presence and reduction of emotional baggage over time as the experienced traveler learns what to leave behind to make traveling easier. Other embedded metaphors might revolve around furniture, such as dressers, or flying on airplanes. You may find other opportunities to launch into "sub-metaphors", depending on your client's needs.

> Now I don't know how you have your clothes organized at home, the ones you keep in your drawers, but you do. And I have a story that maybe you can relate to. This friend of mine was talking about a cousin of hers who likes to travel. When she travels, she likes to buy tee shirts from the various places she visits and bring them back home. Of course, this makes for a fuller bag coming home, which reminds me of the baggage check-in process at airports. Everybody has seen or been through a baggage check at the airport and had their bag checked, all the while noticing other people's bags as well. You know how you notice other people's luggage, how small or large it is, its shape and style, perhaps wondering if the owner is coming or going. And don't we tend to think that when we are departing that all the other folks checking their bags on our flight are also departing, and then when we are returning home, assume that everyone else is also. Then maybe you wonder where they are going to take that piece of luggage: perhaps they will catch a connecting flight that takes them to some destination far away. Did they think about what they would need to take with them, depending on the location, climate, and purpose of the trip? Did they anticipate each day and select particular pieces of clothing, a sort of budgeting? And maybe they divided the days and nights anticipating different needs, selecting particular clothes for each occasion. Who knows what they are taking and what they will bring back.

And when this friend's cousin looks through the drawer in her home that holds her tee shirts that she has collected, she travels all over again. She notices each tee shirt and thinks about where she was when she bought it. She then thinks about the best parts of the visit, maybe a visit to an art gallery, or to a restaurant, or maybe the scenery on a particular tour, you know? She thinks about how she felt and what she learned and she wears all of these tee shirts now and then, selecting carefully, sometimes because she feels a certain way, and sometimes because she wants to. It's interesting how the choice of one or another shirt enhances certain moods and what wearing it may lead to.

Specifically Regretful, Generally Hopeful: Grief Relief

The narrative and language pattern here addresses a process that can be present within the state called regret. Another aspect of the language pattern refers to ingredients that are frequently present in personal problems that lead to distress. We could fairly easily agree that the state of regret refers to some events in our past that we wish had unfolded differently. We may wish we had or had not done or said something—a supposed sin of omission or commission—after which we experience regret. To continue experiencing regret we must essentially place our self in the past, trying to influence events that have ceased to be. Very often a person may find that prolonged regret leads to a feeling of frustration, which is just feedback telling them they have misapplied their focus and energy.

There exists a second essential aspect of regret. As with many other distressing states of emotion, this second aspect seems to be using general principles and applying them to specific events. We make a sweeping generalization and proclaim ourselves to be "bad" or "inconsiderate." But if we examine the details of the past event we may find that we demonstrated numerous traits, some of which we value. Thus, any general labels of self or event can no longer hold water with these exceptions providing the holes. Opportunities are a chance to express a value or achieve some desired outcome. This outcome may be expressing some aspect of our general values or represent a step along the way to some larger goal. An actual experience of an event involves specific ingredients, dynamics, and outcomes. Thus, any and every experience consists of a myriad of pros and cons. We may select which aspects we want to carry forward with us and which we deem "lesson learned", making the necessary adjustments.

Regret often involves focusing on *specifics* of the past, the details, wishing events had happened in a different way. But the present and future hold *general* opportunities to achieve the desired principles. By focusing on the past, the present and future general opportunities pass by, unused. This process seems like looking at the disappearing train that just left the station while missing the next one that's now boarding. The question, "What do you want to happen *now*?" may provide an answer to the frustration of regret. The general and specific principles of the language pattern addressing regret follow.

As you tell me about your concern, I imagine—and you can imagine as well—that I hear that you feel regret and frustration. While this may seem a bit confusing and tangled, you may also look more closely at your regret and frustration and find the same thing. Sometimes people experience an event in a way that they did not want to, things happen that go against a person's values and goals. And when this happens, they may take a look at the specifics of what happened and wonder how it could have turned out differently, how it could have ended the way they wanted. And you know this takes time to do this very important task. And I say this because, if you did not care, you would not review the past, so this task is important. But what may be more important is the *next* task, not reviewing but viewing because all the while, reviewing or viewing, time marches on and change is afoot. And it is this change you want...now. It reminds me of the person who ordered a pizza, you know, decided to eat a pizza, and then decided exactly what ingredients he wanted on this pizza, and then called the pizza place to have it prepared and delivered, and when the pizza delivery person got to his home with the pizza, he had the exact change ready to pay for it. You know how well anticipating coupled with questions works, don't you?

In generally specific terms, you may find that you can extract the general principles from the past and look for an opportunity to use them too...in the present and in the future. Sometimes people miss a friend's birthday and send a card expressing their regret for having missed the birthday, but this happy birthday wish is in the present. And you know a general always outranks a specific, so you can...feel good about knowing that you can use the general for more specific ways, to express and experience this much desired goal now, or maybe you will soon, or maybe in the near future. Or maybe you notice multiple opportunities in the near and nearer as your unconscious mind identifies the general principles that mean so much for you to...utilize and express, while your conscious mind arranges...the specific ways, the pros and cons, goals and purposes to fine-tune this much satisfying. And just how much of this needs to happen for you to know this is different now, as your unconscious mind scans for general opportunities to get specifically meaningful satisfying?...And the energy that comes with this to use now?

Chapter 5
Hypnotic Language Scripts Addressing Perception

This chapter presents and explores the applications of hypnotic language patterns in altering perception. Perception and the Gestalt ingredients that we use to construct our frames play significant roles in creating problems in our daily lives. But this same method of using Gestalt principles to construct frames also may be used differently to create solutions in daily life. The following hypnotic language patterns each address the personal problem by accessing and altering elements of perception and style to create solutions. The first example involves a case of a specific client to better illustrate the process of hypnotic language applied to altering perception. After this, a collection of hypnotic language patterns follows that are tailored to different issues, each relying on altering perception as their point of intervention.

Exploring the Unexplored: Enhancing Perception

This case study utilizing hypnotic language invites the listener to mentally examine a new area: the unmapped territory of the unconscious mind. With an appreciative acknowledgment to Ernest Rossi (2002) as the inventor of the model for this particular intervention, the hypnotherapist here phrases questions in such a way as to invite the listener into the void of unknowing. The phrasing of these questions invites the client into a trance that can then be utilized to identify new resources. The intent is to use questions to help the client move to the outermost edge of conscious awareness, and then just a bit further, into their unconscious mind's unexplored territory.

Distressed clients often present a collection of information gleaned from observations of their past or notions about some dreaded event in the future. The focus is on facts, or imagined facts, and emotions associated with these observations. Clients tend to present this collection of observations and emotions as though the information holds some sort of answer. Such content usually does reveal some answers, but reveals even more how the client handles the problem. A client's presentation through the conscious mind rarely indicates direct solutions to the presenting problem. By probing beyond the conscious stream of problematic events and emotions, however, the client can discover new awareness and thereby effective solutions.

With this perspective in mind, the task of the therapist is to invite the client into unexplored, unimproved territory that is yet to be mapped within the unconscious. Through simple nondirective questioning, the therapist can assist the client to explore new domains. The sequence of this line of open-ended questioning usually proceeds from general to specific bits of information. Of crucial interest here is that the specific bit then leads to another general category of information, the new, unknown territory. The questions concern and select, as the point of conscious mind departure, the bit of information the edge of conscious awareness. This focused question creates a passageway from the conscious mind into the unconscious mind.

The case of Karen will be used as an example of helping the client inspect the previously uninspected portions of her awareness. Karen is a woman in her late thirties. She is married and has two children. Both she and her husband are well-educated, talented people. In Karen's case, she came to counseling for help in dealing with a chronic physical ailment that resulted in much fatigue and physical pain, which resulted in a restricted lifestyle. Karen also ended up working on emotional issues resulting from a tendency to use a passive style in dealing with others.

For the purposes of this example, the focus will be on Karen's emotional distress and dilemmas. Karen's pattern in responding to others is to disconnect from her own wants and needs due to an old value system strongly encouraged by her domineering mother. This value system suggests that Karen must defer to others and give in to them when a difference of opinion occurs. It also suggests that she is to make every effort to keep others happy. As a result, Karen has overextended herself in many ways trying to please others. She holds much pent-up anger that she rarely gives herself permission to express. And finally, Karen has much confusion due to a forgotten process of determining how to know what she wants and feels. Since this maladaptive process is deeply ingrained, we worked in counseling on these issues for several months.

As with most change processes, a stage progression occurs as the person adjusts beliefs, values, and response styles, and then applies these to important areas in life. So it was with Karen. She first began changing how she dealt with her mother, the original source of her misguided values. Sometimes a different order of change takes place, not necessarily starting with the original or most challenging source of one's problems, but this was how Karen changed her life. She did a fine job of setting boundaries and respecting herself while also respecting her mother. This worked well for Karen. After several other pockets of problem areas were adjusted, Karen moved her attention to her home life where, perhaps, the biggest challenge remained.

The challenge at home was for Karen to implement the same strategy as she did with her mother. But at home, she had relationships in the present that held special significance for her with her husband and with her two children. These relationships presented a higher hurdle to overcome than that with her mother. Our goal at that point of therapy was to help Karen reconcile between her needs and the needs of others to find a flexible ability to compromise. The following summary describes the way in which we used hypnotic language to explore the unexplored territory.

The first question I asked Karen was about what she saw when she looked at her personal style at home. "I can't quite tell, it's foggy looking," she responded. I then asked,

> **JB:** So you can't quite see through the fog, huh? You know, sometimes it is foggy and sometimes you hear that the visibility is a quarter of a mile, meaning that you can only see what is a quarter of a mile ahead, and other things beyond this you can only see as a vague outline. And when you walk a quarter-mile ahead, you can see more clearly that what was a half-mile ahead is now a quarter-mile ahead; and what do you see now?

At this point, Karen began noticing how she deferred to others' opinions and others' needs when making choices for herself. She began to notice how she hurt herself by using this decision-making style. She then how she thought and felt she needed to rely on her own needs more in her decision making. She replied, "I need to use my own judgment to decide what's right for me."

I realized that her old style of deferring to others and using their needs as the model for decision making had become habitual, and rather second nature to her. At this point I wanted to help her find a way to recognize her own judgment when it was making itself known to her. With that in mind, I wanted to find an example of a situation when she had relied on her own judgment. In her role as the family "glue", so to speak, the one who holds the family together, I figured she is the one that the family turns to for many decisions and guidance. Ironic, I know, but she was cast in the role of steering the family in many ways. She could decide for others but rarely for herself. I used a common, everyday sort of example of her self-reliant decision making to help her remember how she effectively functions, figuring that Karen would relate to this.

At this point I asked her,

> **JB:** And so how do you know how to tell what you feel versus what others feel? What do you use and how do you know it's yours? [*A pause while she searches.*] In some families, people get some item out of the refrigerator and open it, sniffing and making a funny face. They wonder if the item has gone bad and then ask someone else to sniff.
>
> **Karen:** Yes, we do that in our house too, and I'm the one they ask!

As her voice became more animated I figured she had connected well with this example.

I then asked for details about her way of knowing,

> **JB:** And what do you use to tell you, how do you know? [*Pause while she searches.*]
>
> **Karen:** Well, I know.

In pursuit of details and a deeper awareness of how she knows I asked,

> **JB:** How do you know, what tells you? [*Pause.*]
>
> **Karen:** I use what I know, I feel it, I just know it.

In order to deepen the awareness, I asked,

> **JB:** And this connection to what you know, knowing what you know, how does this feel now?
>
> **Karen:** Strong, good, clear, comfortable.

To generalize to her future I remarked,

> **JB:** And I wonder about all the things you know and all the ways that you can and will use them now and in the future.

We went on to discuss how she can apply this internal "knowing" of hers. She cited several examples with her family and extended family where she could rely on her own judgment and how she would do this. We also discussed various outcome scenarios and some potential reactions by others who might not welcome her new, increased personal strength.

In order to utilize this exploration of the uncharted, unconscious territory, the therapist needs to listen for points in the client's story-telling that indicate uncertainty or fuzziness about resourceful qualities of the self. This includes possible behavior options or times when the client generally reveals some discrepant features in the story or self. This departure from the main theme of feeling stuck may provide an entry into the unconscious. Phrases by the client such as "It's not clear", "It's foggy", "I don't really know", or "I'm not sure", each provide a chance for the therapist to invite the client to explore the unconscious.

The overall key to identifying and using these kinds of statements to explore the unconscious is that the client pauses for an internal search. Uncertainty, pause, and internal search signal a need for more information. In order to experience uncertainty, some degree of competing information must exist. It is this other, yet unexplored and just emerging information that we want to examine. By doing so, the client not only uncovers rich material from the unconscious mind, as Rossi (2002) indicates, but also actually generates new brain cells as the mind accesses and cultivates this new territory.

Follow up with Karen at six weeks and three months revealed that she began and sustained significant self-directed behaviors almost immediately after this session. She initiated a search for resources and combined these to make further changes in her self and her choices according to her own good judgment. These changes led to changes in her relationships within herself as well as within her family. Many family "policy" changes occurred that reportedly brought much greater satisfaction for both Karen and her family.

Determining Frames: Self-Concept

The case presented here concerns the way in which we frame or categorize the information we observe. While the subheading states "determining frames" this conveys two messages with very different meanings. Yes, we categorize information, and the category in which we place the information tends to determine how we respond to situations. But, the other meaning of "determining frames" is that we can consciously determine or *choose* in which category or frame to place information. Thus, we can allow a more resourceful response by building a customized frame.

It seems we categorize information to provide meaning to our observations. But surely we also categorize information in order to organize smaller chunks of information into larger, more manageable general "files". A crucial question in the process of categorizing information is what piece of information is selected from the whole to use as the meaning-making focus. Each event we experience contains a "theme" of sorts.

If you eat at a restaurant or go to a movie, each of these experiences may have a theme. The restaurant or maker of the movie gives this theme, supposedly summarizing the menu or movie content. You may eat at an Italian, Mexican, or vegetarian restaurant. You may watch an action movie, a comedy, or a mystery. Experiences in life get categorized, supposedly based on their most outstanding feature. This most outstanding feature then forms the nucleus of a perceptual gestalt.

It's rather amazing that a single feature of an event can dictate the whole category of an experience. The Italian restaurant also serves a salad with each entrée. So what if the restaurant owner decided to call it a salad restaurant? We can choose what single feature of an event to focus on and then make it the feature of the whole experience. We can also shift from one feature to another, giving a whole new meaning to an experience or event, old or new. And this is where personal power resides—the power to determine the meaning of any event, or change the meaning of any event. Now, this meaning must be believable, not just deception. The meaning must rest on solid, factual evidence, or the category won't be legitimate and positively influential.

To illustrate how this categorizing process functions and dysfunctions, we'll revisit the case of Tony. He came to see me because he was experiencing symptoms of depression as a result of his physical pain and lifestyle restrictions. Tony told me he was really concerned about himself and his abilities. He felt he was losing his mind and going "crazy".

I asked what he meant by this and in what ways he thought this was happening. Tony told me how he'd lately been dropping many things around the house. When he cooked, he'd drop utensils or ingredients. When he was cleaning up around the house, he noticed how he'd drop various items. (I could have pointed out that these mishaps were happening during productive times, thus possibly changing the meaning of the events.) But I believed he would just dismiss the evidence. His sudden perceived increase in dropping things led to him to conclude that he was going "crazy." We could also look at his frame as his feeling that he was losing control in life.

As an intervention strategy I decided to focus strictly on his perceptions and their content. In particular, I relied on the Gestalt perceptual categories of similarities, continuation, and figure-ground. Similarities, as you may recall, refer to our tendency to notice items of a similar nature. Now the theme of this sorting for similarities makes all the difference. You can notice in the room where you are now sitting all items colored blue or green. Or shift to think about categories of boats or indeed any category of items with features in common. In Tony's case, he was noticing the category of things he dropped.

Along with similarities, we also rely on the concept of continuation in this hypnotic language pattern. As described earlier, continuation refers to our tendency to use a perceptual or behavioral theme and just continue utilizing this for each experience. We sort through or respond to situations in the same way, never varying how we process or respond to the information. Continuation resembles the Newtonian principle stating that a body at rest tends to remain at rest, while a body in motion tends to stay in motion. We tend to notice, over time, the same themes or categories. Not only do we notice how items are similar, we *continue* to notice how items are similar. This process tends to illustrate the old phrase, "Everywhere you go, there you are."

The third Gestalt category relied on in this intervention is known as figure-ground. When we perceive a group of information, some part of this group becomes our primary focus (figure), reducing the rest of the group to background material (ground). If you listen to a piece of music played by a band, you could just focus on the piano portion. The piano music becomes the figure, while the music from the other instruments becomes the ground. When we perceive, we usually select some portion of the whole to focus on unless we utilize a more eastern religion mindset of perceiving an undistinguishable whole. Now we revisit the case of Tony as promised earlier, so that we can more fully examine the figure-ground principle. Below is the specific hypnotic language pattern utilized with Tony that resulted from considerable upfront questioning. Following the language pattern is an in-depth discussion about its construction and the principles that were drawn on to construct it.

JB: Tony, I know that you feel as though you are dropping everything you touch. But it may be that this is all you're noticing. Have you ever bought a car, a new car, or just one that's new to you? And as soon as you started on the road to go home you began to notice just how many people have this kind of car. You notice more and more until it seems this is the only kind of car on the road. [*He nods in* *agreement.*] So it may turn out that, just like you didn't notice the cars you didn't notice on the road, there may be many more cars that are different, not similar. So too it may be almost certainly true that you hold on to many more things than you drop. Think about an average day, and just how many things you pick up, and how long you may hold them. Notice how much you pick up and how long you hold it; and just what percentage of the time is this?

To begin the intervention, I asked Tony to think about a general example of similarities sorting. I asked him if he ever noticed after he bought a new car, brand new or just new to him, how he then noticed just how many of the same car and same color there are on the road. Most people can relate to this principle, and so did Tony. Why did I start with addressing his similarities? Well, if you can stop similarities sorting you can stop a particular continuation. I believed Tony was just over-focusing on times when he did drop things. As a result of his focus he'd built a category from stringing these similar "dropping" events together.

I pointed out to him that he can notice all the cars on the road that are similar to his, but in the meantime he's ignoring all the other cars that are different. And which is more? Once he understood this, I applied the perception to his dropping things and wondered if this might also be true for him. I asked him to estimate the percentage of times he drops things compared to the number of times he holds on to things. He naturally found that he held things much more often than he dropped them. Now we have shifted the focal point to the opposite, holding on to things. This shift of focus represents a reversal of figure-ground, switching dropping for holding.

Now we utilize continuation but apply it to holding his new perception in place better. The principle here is that the very same principles that created the problem also create the solution when applied differently. I ask him to think over time about just how many things he has ever picked up and held, choosing only to put them down when he wants to do so. This got him to searching through his memory for like instances, similarity, of holding. Once we collect similar events that are resourceful, we utilize the new focus or figure and then invite continuation to hold this new frame in place. Of course, we need a name for this frame to give it life, so to speak.

I asked Tony what this larger, more enduring perception of his holding things effectively means about him. Tony stated that he guessed he was not "crazy". I then pressed for a specific meaning to take the place of the old. He said his ability to hold things meant he was "O.K." We discussed his meaning of "O.K." and found it was quite a relief for him to realize he was "fine" mentally. Now we can re-visit the incidents of dropping items in the kitchen. This time with a new perceptual lens we find. We considered the fact that these dropping incidents happened in the midst of productive behavior such as cooking and cleaning (meta to the dropping). Tony can place these constructive behaviors within the frame of "O.K.", and "fine," representing factual evidence that these frames about him are were accurate.

I don't want to suggest this example was the only work we did, nor that this simple intervention fully relieved his presented depression. But the collection of principles that go into making frames was called on in various ways over several sessions to dispel and shift his frames from "crazy" and "depressed" to relieving, resourceful frames. Now his physical pain and its life interference no longer adversely affected his mental state. In turn, this no longer exacerbated his physical pain. He knows he can operate from the frames of "O.K." and "fine". At our last session, Tony referred back to the "car principle" and how he continues to remember this idea, finding reassurance about himself through it.

There are several other general principles present in this client's case. I'll highlight them here. First, notice how we each end up relying on the perceptual concepts of deleting, distorting, and generalizing. In order to make a frame, any frame, we utilize this threesome of delete, distort and generalize. But what is its opposite?

Identifying and using opposites of ingredients that construct a frame can lead to deconstructing a frame. Use whatever terms you like to describe the opposite of deleting, distorting, and generalizing. I use *including*, *factualizing*, and *specifying*. The process of including more information into awareness defeats deleting, the process of factualizing defeats distorting, and the process of specifying defeats generalizing. Think about it and notice the difference.

The second principle expressed in this case is what amounts to the gestalt of frames. Each frame consists of a gestalt made up of information with a focal point or theme. This frame theme holds the frame together and further relies on such Gestalt perceptual principles as similarities, continuation, simplification, closure, and figure-ground to maintain itself.

These perceptual principles greatly influence what we observe, how we observe it, and what meaning we give our observations. So a frame results from a gestalt, or whole. This whole stems from a particular focus on a particular item or group, thus defining the frame. What drives us to select the particular object or subject of our focus is a whole other matter. What is important is that we can intervene and choose to make our own frames, thus creating the experiences and meanings of our lives.

Rejecting Transplants: Resistance

The purpose of this story is to address the apparent natural tendency we each possess to resist change or resist ways that are new to us. I liken this mental resistance process to the body's natural defense system that automatically rejects a transplanted organ just on principle. The immune system has to be suppressed in order for the body to finally realize that the new part will benefit the person.

It seems clients I've worked with and maybe people in general go through some sort of change preparation stages prior to implementing actual personal change. This initial phase may appear as some form of resistance. "Resistance" more often seems to result from the counselor not assessing the individual's dynamics sufficiently. The counselor may not account for the client's concerns about the consequences of the upcoming change. But even with assessing the client, each individual seems to necessarily negotiate the change process, coming to rest in a new style of thinking, emoting, and behaving.

I believe that we possess a mental immune system that acts similarly to the physical immune system, defending and protecting the status quo. This mental immune system with its defense mechanisms—different from Freud's defense mechanisms—lacks foresight and so reacts automatically to any suggestion of a new mental set that might require altering the cognitive-perceptual style and belief system of the individual. The defense mechanisms of our mental immune system do not rely on the defense mechanisms identified by Freud, which tend to become activated in response to some imagined outside threat.

These mental immune system defense mechanisms that I refer to are internal and more primitive. They fight change for the sake of fighting change, as part of a basic principle that motivates the mental–emotional system to maintain itself and resist change. It seems this immune system reacts to a change in cognitive-perceptual and belief systems as the physical immune system reacts to an organ transplant, rejecting this apparent intruder just because it's foreign. However, developing and communicating new ways to use old defenses can convert an enemy into an ally. It seems there exists a positive correlation between the degree of emotional injury and the strength of the immune system's resistance to change. The therapist's positive regard and respect for the client's much-needed sense of safety gained by the mental immune system can go a long way toward creating a safe atmosphere for positive change.

The following language pattern is designed to be applied in the case of a client who tends to self-defeat due to some negative belief about self that acts as a defense mechanism at some primitive level of thinking. But in the effort to change oneself, this same mechanism holds the individual hostage.

This was a movie script that I read once, or maybe twice, I don't remember, and I don't even remember if it was ever made into a movie. You know lots of scripts are not made into movies. Anyway, the story revolves around the military defense system known as Star Wars. The orbiting system shoots down any nuclear missiles in flight. Well, one day a group of astronomers, you know the scientists who look way out into space and find planets...they sometimes find "new" planets, but the planet is not really new, it is just noticed for the first time. The astronomers who were looking through the telescope saw a huge meteor out in space. The meteor must have looked really tiny through the lens of that big telescope, so the scientists had to figure out how they knew that even though it looked tiny, it was really very big. Kind of like how things in the distance look really small but we have a way of figuring out and knowing how big they really are. And this ratio of the size of an object and its distance from us, the further the smaller, is sort of like our future and maybe how we don't take it seriously enough. Our distant future looks so small that maybe we ignore it or disregard it. But then it gets closer and bigger, and we find out that we have ignored it for too long.

Well, these astronomers saw this really big meteor. They could also tell it was headed for Earth. And they knew by its size that it would do great damage if it hit the Earth. Some scientists think that the ice age happened because a huge meteor hit the earth and caused a huge, thick dust cloud to surround the earth, making for extremely cold weather for a long time, freezing out and killing many things.

Well, the astronomers knew for sure this meteor would hit the Earth and they had to figure out some way to destroy it. They sure could not move the Earth out of its way. So experts got together from many countries to put their fine minds together and think of ways to destroy the meteor and save Earth. These experts were from a variety of countries and cultures. Some knew each other and had worked together before. And some knew each other but had been enemies. But now, with this common cause, they united in their work to find a solution.

And while they each had differing relationships from the past, they were surprised to find out such new and interesting things now. Each provided some useful and beneficial input that led to the final solution. In the process of working out this solution, each expert came to know, really know, the person they worked with as a person and not as an expert from some particular part of the world. They found they had so much in common and old concepts just melted away, leading to new and very powerful bonds of supportive and understanding friendship.

So these experts came together and worked together and discovered all this surprising and interesting information about each other. This in the midst of finding a solution to the impending disaster, they finally decided that they had better get to work on putting a plan into action or all these new friendships would perish. This group of experts decided the best way would be to shoot several nuclear missiles at the meteor while it was still a good distance away from earth. This would blow up the meteor and scatter it away from Earth.

They got other nations with such destructive weapons to agree to each fire several missiles to destroy the meteor. They fired one at a time, since the follow-up shots would need to be based on the new location of the pieces of the meteor that were left after each successive blast, the biggest and most threatening pieces would be shot at first.

Now timing was crucial, so they had to wait to fire the missile until the meteor was close enough to hit. One nation fired off its nuclear missile. It was on its way up and to the edge of the atmosphere, making a beeline for the meteor. All of a sudden, the Star Wars technology system went into action. It fired one of its own missiles and did just as it was designed to do; it destroyed a nuclear missile in flight. Whoa! Who was prepared for this?

Now another country fired its missile just in case the first was a fluke. On its way toward the meteor at the edge of the atmosphere and BOOM! the Star Wars system strikes again and obliterates the nuclear missile. Oh no! Soon it became apparent that the good people of Earth were trapped by their own invention, their defense system now prevented them from defending themselves. How ironic it all seemed. Now these great scientists, who thought they had figured out a certain solution, found themselves stuck. They were not sure now what to do or what to use to try to stop the meteor from obliterating Earth. Time was passing and the meteor was getting closer at a very fast rate of speed. Finally, after much worry, pressure, and anxiety, the scientists decided to talk to the designers of the Star Wars system.

What they found out was amazing! The system was on a sort of auto-pilot so that it would just automatically shoot down any missiles in flight. At first this seemed like such a design would surely doom them all. But the designers of the Star Wars system began thinking about their design. They realized that if the system had once been set up in one way, it could also be set up in another way.

The Star Wars' designers accessed the setting of their system and adjusted the setting. Now a newer and even more effective design became activated. The new defense system missiles could be aimed at the incoming meteor and treat it as if it were a nuclear missile. Not only this but the number of missiles fired could also be adjusted so that only the number really necessary to do the job would be fired off. Once this adjustment was complete, the scientists activated it.

Almost instantly, the Star Wars system readjusted itself and took aim at the meteor. The missile arsenal closest to the meteor fired a missile and immediately hit its target. The meteor was impacted and began breaking apart. The orbiting missile system then picked out the next biggest piece and fired directly at it, shattering it in so many small pieces that they would just harmlessly burn up while entering the Earth's atmosphere, disappearing completely. This process continued another time or two as needed. Now, what had been a huge meteor heading straight for Earth became a very small collection of pieces. Some of these pieces were bypassing Earth, totally out of awareness. And the others just harmlessly burned up into pure vapor, vanishing completely. What a redesign! Taking many factors into account so that what was threatening was removed and what was preserving remained.

Refueling: Knowing the Sources of Well-Being

This language pattern seeks to help the listener shift from an external source of life energy to one within the self, and then to an ultimate source, the universal source and flow of energy. Only use this pattern for those clients who hold such concepts as a universal source and flow of energy. I have used this pattern with people of differing persuasions, such as agnostics and Christians, with equally beneficial results. You may or may not agree with this concept of a universal oneness, but the hypnotic process in this pattern can be very helpful in gaining access to an unlimited energy source.

I use the metaphor of military airplanes that require fuel in flight and air tankers that provide the fuel to metaphorically convey the limitations of self as the source of life energy. Why military planes? It seems that people who rely on others as their fuel source, or even those who feel they must pull their own load in isolation easily become defensive and self-protective due to such a precarious arrangement. Maybe their past experiences and resulting defensiveness led them to choose going it alone. Either way, this metaphor then allows addressing self-defense, protection, and felt vulnerability and intends to shift the listener to a safer source of fuel. The solution suggested in the metaphor comes from converting a provider of fuel into a perpetual receiver of fuel that can then utilize this fuel to perform better.

This is an interesting story that I'm going to share with you. Now, you may or may not be a fan of science fiction, as opposed to science fact, but nonetheless, please listen and consider the story because you know that most of science fiction is really just a vehicle to carry some other sort of message disguised within the story.

Now, this particular story concerns an airplane, a military airplane. This airplane is from the recent past, well who's to decide how recent recent is? But this plane was quite advanced in many ways, an advanced plane. It could fly very fast and could maneuver with incredible precision. All the pilots wanted to fly it, but only a few were specially trained to be able to fly such a fast and highly maneuverable airplane. The pilots would just zoom through the air at great speeds doing all kinds of precise maneuvers. While this plane was really, really fast and could loop and turn and turn with amazing grace, one problem plagued it…fuel. This plane was sort of like a cheetah. It could go really fast and move with great precision but only for a short time. So the military faced a problem in that this plane was designed to keep people safe, it could only do so for a short time, leaving people vulnerable again. The military then decided to figure out how to develop a plane that would be specially made just to carry fuel. This was a tanker plane, filled with special jet fuel. This tanker plane also had a special device that acted like a fuel pump. This tanker plane was a flying gas station for the high-speed military plane. Maybe you've seen film footage of planes refueling in mid-flight. The small plane maneuvers ever so carefully up to the tanker plane. The tanker plane has its fuel nozzle ready and the two link up to re-fill the small plane.

Now this helped, but only to an extent. This really, really fast and maneuverable jet could fly longer, but was still dependent on the tanker plane to keep flying beyond a short time or distance. So the military was still limited and sort of stuck. Then creativity happened. What if this special plane had built into it a device that could convert naturally occurring forces into fuel, so that it could develop perpetual motion? Yes, but great but how and what? What if some constant external source could be brought within and converted into fuel? Wow, now this suggested true independence! The military minds thought and thought and they brought in some very creative people to help them find a solution: finding and converting an external source into internal fuel that would permit flying at will…imagine this…flying at will.

Well now these creative people had it, an idea. This creative team just did some very simple thinking really, identifying already existing sources that could be converted into internal energy sources, sun, and wind. Solar panels along the body of the plane can take in the energy from the sun and convert it into fuel that powers the engine. And maybe even more clever, or at least a companion idea that kicks it up a notch: windmills of sorts in the wings that convert the moving air while in flight into perpetual energy to fuel the plane as long as it wants to move.

Now the plane did not have to supply or seek fuel supplies, dependent on another source. This plane can convert the raw energy that's always available into energy that fuels its flights that can allow freedom of motion and range. It became an interesting experience for the pilots of this new, self-sufficient plane. They could feel the quantum leap from the old way of having to get fuel put inside from the outside to the new, way of making energy from the inside from a limitless, boundless, infinite source of energy within.

And thinking about the difference, looking and feeling within, allow yourself to find and know this internal, eternal receiving source inside you. [*Pause while the client searches.*] And as you feel…within… Finding   feeling…connecting with this receiving source of yours just let me know when you know you have this awareness and connection fully. You can just gently nod your head when you know and feel this is established clearly and fully… [*Pause until the client gives this or some other established ideomotor signal. The head nod is just an option. You can use a finger signal or any other ideomotor form of communicating.*] And now notice and feel this fuel, absorbing and enjoying this effortless filling…and the many ways you can use as you choose.

False Sense and Self-Reliance

One of the most significant shifts that take place within our self as we negotiate our way through various developmental levels is the pivotal move from relying on an external locus of control to an internal locus. When we transfer our ways of knowing from things and people outside of self to our own internal awareness, we necessarily rely on our own senses, perceptions, thoughts, and emotions. This re-arranging of how we relate with others can change the roles and purposes of relationships. This change often results in interesting dynamics within self and between self and others.

The change from external locus to internal locus can expose a toxic relationship. I say this because many clients that I work with—perhaps you as well—find that when they shift from external to internal locus, those who had manipulated them emotionally or used them in some way begin objecting to the changes. And one of the crucial ways someone maintains emotional or behavioral manipulation of another is by suggesting that the controlled person doubt their senses. They should doubt what they think, believe, and sense. If the manipulator can implant enough doubt in the other, then control opportunities remain available. Very often, when a child is growing up and attempting to negotiate a stage of development that involves increasing autonomy or individuation, the controller will attempt to exert influence here.

This influence often comes in a form that subtly or overtly suggests that the developing individual doubt what they know; thus remaining in the controller's emotional clutches. While this battle for control continues, the younger one maintains natural needs for advancement and expanding their sphere of influence, their individuation. The needs continue yet the child is told their needs are wrong.

This discrepancy between needs and teachings then sets up an approach–avoidance conflict. The child wants to approach new stimuli and situations but has been told to avoid them. They may then develop beliefs that tell them they should not want what they naturally want, personal development. The result of this dilemma can play out as extensive, repeated self-defeating behavior or personal stagnation. The child then comes to blame themselves for their decisions when they are really the result of this toxic loyalty that stymies development.

The following hypnotic language pattern addresses this crucial set of dynamics, influences, decisions, and consequences. Adjust the gender of the main character of the story to match that of your client.

> Once upon a time, which is a sort of interesting concept when you stop to think about this traditional line that we hear introducing so many stories from childhood. Once upon a time? We reside upon time and ride it? Hmmm, once upon a time. Just what does this mean and how do we hear it here and think about it when we stop

and really think? Well, anyway, once upon a time there was this woman, actually she started out as a girl, and so this is where and when the story starts.

She was a girl who lived on an island, really a young woman but sort of still a girl as well. She was being raised by her mother and father. Now her father was a hard-working man who spent much time working for many hours at a time, putting in long days. While he did this and provided for his family, his wife, the girl's mother, was in charge of raising her. Her mother was a very strict woman who wouldn't put up with any nonsense.

This small island was pleasant enough, with many trees, a water view as all islands have, and plenty of food to eat if they were careful and both grew their own food and hunted for more. This island had only one real road. I call it a road, but it was more a wide, smooth path that was easy to walk. This lone road went all the way around the island, a big loop. No matter at what point you got on the road, you could always tour the whole island and end up where you started, simple and yet very predictable, limited to the island.

There were also some other people who lived on this island. And these people were known to this girl, since everybody knew everybody else, at least to some extent. You could not really avoid contact with others, which was good for a little variety and some change of pace really. But the routine and variety soon became known and then there was really very little if any variety. The weather came to provide the most variety, but even this was fairly predictable. However, there were some interesting events that happened from time to time involving other people and their families who lived on the island.

The island was not really that far from another island and this island was fairly near the mainland. There was a bridge that linked this island to the second island and another bridge linking the second island to the mainland. The first bridge was a sort of suspension bridge made of wood and rope, making it rather unsteady and unstable, easily swaying over the churning water below. In fact, the word was that you could not really trust this first bridge and that it would not support a person crossing it. Rumor had it that the second bridge was quite stable and secure, but that no one knew for sure, since no one had ever really crossed the first bridge. For this very reason, at the shore just under the first bridge, there was a designated rescue team. This team was equipped with two boats to rescue anyone who might try to cross the bridge and fall off into the water. This girl who lived on the island was told many times by her mother that this bridge was unsafe and that, if she ever tried to cross it, she would fall helplessly into the water and drown.

Curiosity being what it is, allowing each to search, pursue, and learn, she decided to walk to the bridge and just sit there to watch anyone who might try to cross. At first she felt nervous just walking to the bridge, her mother's warning ringing in her ears. She reached the bridge, hearing the water below and there was no one in sight. She stood motionless for a few minutes, feeling her fear. Then, since she knew she was not even going to try to cross it, she sat and decided to watch. Yet deep within herself she could feel the wonder and longing to know. She kept this down within and just watched.

The first day she watched as a young man approached the bridge, attempting to cross. But as he began crossing, her heart racing in her chest, she saw the bridge begin to sway. The further he walked along the bridge, the more it swayed and soon, fearing the bridge would collapse, he just leaped off the bridge into the water, at just about the halfway point of the bridge. He yelled as he leaped and fell into the water. The rescue team scrambled to their boat and instantly launched out into the water. They made their way to this scared and foundering young man, helping him into the boat, and took him back to shore.

Even from where she sat watching, this girl could feel the stark terror of this rescued young man. No one else attempted to cross the bridge this day. But the next day, taking up her observation position again, another young person, this time a girl, approached the bridge. This girl approached the bridge, paused, and then continued walking onto the bridge. The swaying began immediately and yet she continued walking. As she progressed, the swaying got worse and worse. Now the walker and the observer each felt such great fear. The girl on the bridge leaped off and into the water just before she reached the halfway point. Again the rescue team activated and swiftly moved out into the water, scooping up the terrified girl. The girl observing sat in awe, feeling the fear that she had been told was real.

Deep within her, though, deeper than the current in the water below, began a stirring, a longing, an awareness of an empty, unfulfilled need. Yes, she had watched as the bridge fulfilled its reputation. And yes, she'd seen how the people attempting to walk across had finally had enough and jumped into the water, been rescued, and returned to the island. But she knew there was more to this and she knew that she had to know what it was.

As she began thinking, playing the sequence of events from her past to these most recent events, she took careful stock of the ingredients and the parts, players in all. Some things appear to be a set, a sort of prearranged match. The trees and the fruit they bear. The soil and the crops it grows. The rain, the sunshine, and the crops they nurture. Then while looking at the bridge, she began to sort of separate and dissect the parts, wondering how it got this way and was this the only way things could be arranged and if these were the only ingredients that could be used and just how many ingredients and how many ways could the various ingredients work together.

At this moment, this very precise moment, she suddenly realized, looking down below, she saw the boat. Now this was just electrifying her mind. Yes, the bridge is the great, feared, unstable, unreliable bridge. But what had she seen each time that was reliable? In the process of the turmoil, she'd seen this rescue boat go out into the water, rough water at that, and do its task safely. Well, if this boat can go out halfway across the water and then come back to the island shore, this same boat can cover the same total distance in a straight line, moving it all the way across to the other side. What new territory this opened up. This boat had already proven itself seaworthy; and she had seen this for herself. She had also seen exactly how the boat is operated and the way to maneuver it through the water. It is as though she had been in school for this and it was now time to use what she'd learned.

She now knew exactly how to come and go as she pleased. Carefully making her way down to the unused boat, she boarded it and made her way across the water to the other side, knowing exactly how to do this. Such freedom as she moved. So exhilarating as she reached the other side, scrambling up the shore to find the next bridge and to further freedom she moved. Sure enough, she found the next bridge that proved much more secure, barely questioning, just noticing how to navigate her way across. She made her way to the mainland and all it had to offer. Now rarely returning to her island of origin. So much has changed and so much had remained the same. The gap between and the chosen position seem to be the biggest matter. Decisions based on faulty, imposed beliefs that were only held out of loyalty and trust. How can we cross a bridge made of materials from another who proves untrustworthy? The materials will not support us by design. We will fall through, as they intend. What methods do you know of that you already really know and know how to use now, haven't you and will again?

Dissociating

The collection of hypnotic language patterns presented below consists of ways to dissociate from a problem or limiting belief. During the course of therapy, one of the essential steps in healthy change includes disconnecting or dissociating from the problem. This disconnecting or dissociating includes separating from the problematic perceptual level, thought patterns, gestalt formation and, ultimately, beliefs and states. In the process of therapy you might find that you first identify the issue needing a change and then begin presenting examples of ways the client can dissociate. Once dissociated from the old problematic issue and the accompanying perceptual–cognitive aspects, you can then examine and establish new ways of perceiving and thinking to allow new meaning about old circumstances.

Through the Surface: Dissociating

The hypnotic pattern below is designed to help the client dissociate or step back from current experience. The metaphor used involves water: perhaps a lake or some smooth body of water. If you've ever looked at the surface of a lake when the water was especially smooth, you may have noticed that there are two distinct views available, the mirror like surface reflecting the sky above and the view of what is below the surface of the water. This dichotomy provides a good example representing the conscious and unconscious minds, the reflected sky and what resides below the water's surface, respectively. If you like, you could just as easily let the metaphor use the water's surface as the conscious and then invite the client to focus on the *reflected* image and go up into the clouds above by looking at the water below. Hypnotic already isn't it? Either way you like, you can help the client dissociate through this metaphor, with or without the entry point about fishing.

Toward the end of the pattern, there is a reference to the biblical story of the loaves and fishes. Certainly you can either use this portion with a client who you know is of the Christian faith or just leave it out. The purpose of utilizing the miracle of the loaves and fishes is to establish a state of comfort and lasting reassurance while otherwise dissociated. But you can establish states of lasting comfort in many ways, without drawing on the loaves and fishes story. Either way, you can then utilize the client's dissociated state to introduce other informative processes and metaphors to this heightened state of receptivity.

You know, everybody knows what fishing is. Maybe you've gone fishing before or know someone who has, or maybe you've even seen someone fishing on TV or in a movie. This person who is fishing, at some point, gets into their boat while it is at the shore, then pushes off, maybe with a paddle or maybe by starting the engine and glides along the water, moving away from the shore further out onto the lake. Somehow, this fisherman decides just where to come to rest and just float and fish. Maybe he knows of a particular spot for the best fishing or maybe he just goes by feel, you know, sort of senses where he thinks the best catches will be. He prepares, casts, and then waits, just watching the water. And when you think about this body of water you can notice that the surface of the water reflects the sky. You can look down to look up and see the sky with whatever clouds may be there. And if you look long enough you can even see the clouds drift across the water, but you know it's really in the sky. And if you look a bit more you can just start ignoring those clouds and begin looking through the surface of the water and start seeing beneath the surface. Maybe you just see a few particles and then maybe you see a fish. You can watch the fish drift and swim and notice the scales and fins of this fish as it moves through the water.

And then you can look where the fish is not, and just notice the water. If you look a bit deeper, you may be able to see something else, noticing at first a small movement and then seeing the outline, gradually filling in the details of another fish. And then you can look where this fish is not and maybe see just the water beneath the surface. And then another fish comes into view. This collection of fish may remind you of just how many fish, and how many kinds of fish exist. And this may remind you of other things that you think about when you think about fish.

Maybe you begin to remember the wonderful miracle of the loaves and fishes when Christ performed this for the people who were hungry. How Christ drew upon the infinite that is, infinitely, and bringing this here for people to benefit from and the infinite comfort knowing this can provide.

And your conscious mind can remember and enjoy this awareness while you unconscious mind thinks about all the ways to enjoy this. Or maybe your unconscious mind just continues enjoying this awareness and feeling, while your conscious mind feels the benefit. All the while, either way, you can find and feel this much more comfort and reassurance.

Student-Teaching: Dissociating

This pattern is simply used to help the client dissociate from old, limiting beliefs, perceptions, and/or behaviors. The reasoning for helping the client dissociate from old patterns is to shift the client from living from in a restricted way to reclaiming freedom of choice. A crucial step in the process of change is disconnecting from old styles. This language pattern uses the metaphor of a school building and classrooms to aid in the disconnecting process. The school building is also used to help the client step back in time to a point in childhood when perhaps they learned these limiting styles. Essentially, the client is first associated into the old mindset and time, and then helped to disconnect from the old permitting new connections and styles.

Every town has buildings and everyone has seen various types of buildings of various sizes, and shapes. And some buildings are just one storey high, while others are multiple stories. Just about all buildings have some windows in them, allowing those outside to look in and those inside to look out. And it can be interesting to be outside looking in and wonder just what it looks like on the inside, then going in to find out. Once in you may find various rooms and then each room has a particular size, depending on the purpose of the room. In particular, one type of building, called a school, has room for learning.

You know everybody has been a student at one time or another. And some have even taught, including you. And it can be a very interesting experience, depending on where you are in the room. Maybe you were sitting at the back of the room, looking at all the other students, or maybe you were off to one side or another, noticing how things looked from there. You may see the desk you're in, and notice details, maybe it was a flat or a slanted desk, maybe with a wooden seat. And then you may notice other students' desks. And thinking about these, you notice how they vary. Or maybe you were up at the front of the room, in your seat. Then again, maybe you were the teacher or trainer. Depending on the position, the many looking at the one, or the one looking at the many and all you see.

And all this takes place in just one setting, not sitting. Thinking now about all the other classes, students, rooms, and subjects one to many ideas, since so many ideas are taught, you know. And maybe you drift back to a particular time when you learned something very valuable, or maybe you drift back to a person who taught you and this was so valuable. Or maybe your conscious mind just sort of imagines a collective experience of learning and then knowing. Perhaps your unconscious, capable of so much more knowing how to sort and find all the particular learning experiences, then passing them, as needed to your conscious. And as you think about thinking, because you know you have to think to learn, you can just find this much more security and comfort as you go deeper, then deepest knowledge provides...this now as you come across this most fine certainty. And learning is both a conscious and an unconscious process. Just like you learned how to learn the multiplication tables and dedicated them to memory. So you can think about specific learnings or some general category of learnings, or the collective lifetime of learnings and continue to find even more...skill and comfort in this.

Anyway you like, you can continue knowing you possess much knowing that continues growing *your* skills and comfort so that your unconscious mind finds and feels this, while your conscious mind experiences the many benefits. And even while you continue learning new things, you can know that you know how to learn, utilizing this wonderful learning ability to learn and master new skills, to add to your collection and the feelings this brings. Using what you learn or learning what you use that works so well. And in a way, to access what you have learned and know, you disconnect from the moment, step away and search, finding what it is you know you want to remember...how to use this.

Taking Note: Dissociating

This pattern might well serve someone in high school or college, or someone with an issue stemming from that developmental period.

The purpose of the pattern is to help the listener dissociate from current emotional states, thoughts, and beliefs in order to access more effective resources. The pattern is a lead into dissociating, which may then set the stage for additional hypnosis or hypnotic language that leads to solutions for the client.

> Have you ever been writing, taking notes in a class and noticed your pen or pencil moving across the paper, leaving a trail. And then…[*Pause*]…looking over at a friend taking notes and notice…their pen or pencil, while it's the same in some ways, it looks different just because it's not your own and yet it may be making some the very same words you made with yours, separate yet the same. Or when you're sitting in a room, maybe a waiting room…and you're tired of waiting, ready for change, and you notice your shoes, the color and shape. And then you notice the shoes of the person next to you and imagine that these are your shoes. It's funny how things look different when they belong to you and they belong to someone else. And how often do you think about whether or not your shoe laces are tied? …Yes, and then you immediately fix this, don't you, at the first chance you get…right?

Ways of Forgetting: Perception Shifts

Sometimes in the course of counseling, the client needs to learn how to leave behind some old, ineffective, or even detrimental beliefs, memories, or behavioral styles. They need to learn a different way and remember how to forget the old, leaving behind limiting aspects of self. Hypnotic language can provide an effective way to help the client forget what needs to be forgotten.

The following collection of hypnotic language patterns attempts to utilize metaphors to convey ways of forgetting. This category of hypnotic language equates to moving the old frame into a new frame, giving it new meaning and influence, or lack of influence. The process involves finding a new, more desirable category in which to store the old information, one that will achieve the goal. In the process of delivering the hypnotic language, you access and activate the new category or frame by making repeated reference to examples of this category. Once the new category, in this case forgetting, is established through repeated examples, then refer to the old information, linking it with the new category. You may also find that these patterns help the client to dissociate not just from a particular memory but also to dissociate in general. These patterns may be useful in whole, as they are written, or you may find that just certain parts you select and string together work well.

Defogging the Windshield

Now, you know everybody has had the experience when they were driving, or maybe you were a passenger, and the car window fogs up, really limiting your vision. If the fog is on the inside, maybe you decide to write something in the fog. And you know there are two general ways to leave your mark: either you can mark on a clean slate, which then shows up, or you can remove certain parts of a full slate, revealing information in the gaps. And in the case of the fogged windshield, the car has a setting on the instrument panel that is usually marked "Defrost". Now does this mean it will only work when there is frost? And will it work if it is liquid, not frozen, as well? No and yes. So you may remember using this setting when the windshield was fogged, setting the temperature of the air that flows out and setting the dial to guide the air to come out at just the right place to achieve the goal. Once on, you can even hear it. And then this rather intriguing process happens that can be fascinating to watch, almost mesmerizing. You may choose to look at just the very bottom tip of the fog as the air comes out at just the right temperature, and you can see the fog begin to disappear. It just seems to roll up the windshield. Your eyes can follow it, and watch as it continues rolling and once it starts it just gets faster and faster until...poof...it's gone...vanished...evaporated...revealing such clear vision that you can see what is right in front of you so clearly.

Scent Away

Maybe at some time or another, like most people, you have found yourself at the cologne or perfume counter in a department store. Maybe you were shopping for yourself or maybe you were shopping for someone else. And even if you had as your main goal, sampling and buying a scent, you might find yourself looking at some other things throughout the store. You know, you can look at one thing and then maybe another, but all the while you can know, and even feel, this agenda, this unfinished, unsatisfied yet-to-be-done mission. So you move about the store, looking, touching, feeling, as you make you way to the scents. And even before you get right up to the counter, before you come to your scents, you can begin to notice the faint scents of these perfumes or colognes. And maybe you have a particular one you want to sample, try on. Or maybe you have a particular brand you want to sample. And so, with highest eagerness and anticipation, you try on the first one, inhaling carefully and feeling how it smells. Which is kind of interesting, asking our self how we feel about a smell. We never ask our self how a feeling smells, do we? Well, maybe getting hurt stinks. So you sample and try on some different scents in different ways and different spots. At first the scent is clear. And you can even differentiate the first from the second. But, by the third and, for sure, the fourth, you begin to lose the ability to tell the difference and they seem to begin to blend into one and then none, searching for what is no longer there and yet missing nothing. Have you ever noticed how, when you first smell a particular scent, it seems very noticeable? It stands out. But, after awhile, this scent gradually diminishes, and actually fades from your awareness until you don't even notice it at all? In fact, you even forgot how it was that it did smell…vanished, returning to the original clear scent sending you on your way to where you next want to go and this fresh start.

Forgetting and Not Noticing: Letting Go of Limits

The following collection of patterns emphasizes ways to forget. The language pattern guides the listener into accessing the category of things we forget and, even more, things we do not notice to begin with. By accessing these categories, the client can then transfer what they want to forget into this category where things are forgotten. The purpose of letting go of limiting memories is to allow the client to move forward into creating a desired future.

There are some things that we each forget. Sometimes we forget because we want to and sometimes we forget though we do not want to. So regardless of why we forget, it is interesting to notice that each of these instances can have a variety of effects.

I was listening to a friend tell me about her recent experience and she said she had not felt so relaxed since she did not remember when…she felt so relaxed by forgetting everything else and just remembering this relaxing feeling. So you know you can forget and just relax.

And sometimes we don't necessarily forget, we just never notice, so we never knew we never knew …You don't notice what's not in the grocery store. You didn't notice the cars you didn't notice on the road today, let alone yesterday and tomorrow. And you can go right on not noticing what is not there. Just like when you may have looked at another car on the road as you rode, and saw the car and the driver and maybe there were some passengers in the car, or not. But you did not notice who was not in the car, and you can keep on not noticing what is not here or there. In fact, you've forgotten many things in your life so well that you don't remember that you forgot. You may not remember the last time you used the number 462, and you may not even remember the time before that, having forgotten completely. I overheard in the hallway one time, and I forget where now…just ignore what you want to forget.

And everyone's had the experience of trying to remember something. And they just about recall, it gets to the tip of their tongue, and they try and try unsuccessfully to remember and then they just say, "Oh, forget it," and they do. And you can think about or try to think about the things you've forgotten, maybe some old math formula or some foreign language words, but can't really remember because you forgot. And maybe it's just your conscious mind that can't remember or perhaps it's your unconscious mind that forgets. But you can remember to forget or forget to remember, and it's just as well, since you can trust your unconscious to know what to forget and remember to do this so that, as your conscious mind does without, not even knowing what it doesn't know, and it's odd even while your unconscious mind deletes permanently what it knows it can forget, which means you can now as well."

I like to use metaphors and hypnotic language, so I'll use some here and you may wonder just when this one begins, but then you'd have to leave here and begin searching through the past but you'd be better off hearing here now because this is what's happening and holds the answers to your future, your present, so open up to experience your present, now didn't you? Find what and how…to really listen now and focus on the immediate present so you can…better utilize this now.

Now you may remember the first day of kindergarten or first grade and maybe the last day of kindergarten or first grade. And you may remember some other first days of the school year and you may remember some other last days of the school year but you forgot everything in between. And now you can think about a feeling of deep comfort…and the one before this…and the next one coming and forget about everything else in between so that you just have this sense of a series of comfortable feelings linking one to the next to the next comfortable feeling.

Sometimes you forget something because you no longer need to know. Think about words that we no longer use and of course you can't because we and you no longer use them, so you can just continue forgetting because the situation no longer exists. The word "pop-top" no longer gets used because pop-tops no longer exist. We threw that term away just like we did pop-tops. And just like some words cease because the situation no longer exists, some words get created because a situation is new and different like fax. This new word, fax, that came…to exist because of a new condition or situation…just the present facts.

And the whole time that I've been talking and you've been listening and thinking, you never once thought about a bee sting. [*In general, cite an example of an activity associated with an undesirable experience or undesirable state of emotion*] and you never once thought about the highest praise you ever received. [*Choose an example of a desirable experience or state of emotion*] …the difference…between the two…tells you which to forget…and which to remember, which is desirable.

Icebreaker: Arthritis

The metaphor presented in this story is designed to address the symptoms and process of arthritis. The story moves from problem to resolution, with the idea that it parallels the process of arthritis, and then provides a solution. After the client goes into a moderately deep trance through whatever means you choose, present the following story.

As you feel this deepest sense of relaxation flow through you, I want to tell you about another flow, that of a river. This story involves a really large river, one so large that it carries much boat traffic on it, from cargo ships to recreational and pleasure boats. These vessels travel up and down this large flowing river for many purposes. And one winter the weather was especially cold and the river froze. It froze so quickly and so solidly that many of the boats on the river were stuck, literally in midstream. Well, the passengers and crews and captains of these vessels were really frustrated and felt angry at being stuck. They knew where they came from and where they wanted to go but just could not budge their vessels. Not only were these people angry, but they also felt some worry about their situation. When and how would it be settled?

This extreme locking up of the river was a once-in-a-lifetime happening and was surely temporary. The seasoned river folk knew that they had only to wait while the air warmed, heating and thawing the river. They also knew that the water beneath the ice was warmer and would eventually work its way up as the warmth began melting the ice from above. As the sun came out, they could see the steam begin to rise from the ice, a sure sign of thawing. They could watch the steam rise and notice the ice changing hue as it melted further. The ice went from a clear, hard, stiff solid white to a sort of cloudy, softening mass that eventually became a mush. And as this mush warmed even more it began to separate and move apart, exposing warmer water.

The sun continued shining, providing additional warmth as it climbed higher in the sky. The ice really was not ice any more, rather it was a soft mush that began to merge with the warmer waters, warming even more. Soon the captains could feel their ships begin to move, first just slight bobs and gentle motions. Then more room to move became available as what was ice now simply became water, integrating with only a few, shrinking pieces melting quickly.

Forward motion returned to the ships and they could now power themselves in their chosen direction, some going upriver, and some going downriver. Relief filled each person as each boat moved freely, floating and flowing as all vessels, from cargo to recreational to pleasure boats now easily float freely, moving as they need to where they need and want to go now. And as they flow on the river they watch the warming waters gently glide by. They notice how deep the waters run and take great comfort from the depth of the support, deeper than they know. They think about this and look forward to future times on the river while enjoying this one as well. This sense of the river always being present, even in the future, provides comfort and security for all passengers.

And no matter what happens from this point to the future, with your now freely flowing movements, you can...as your conscious mind may wonder when and how this too will happen, that your unconscious what can simply, show the conscious mind what it knows and then the rest...you will know as well.

Out of Context: Comparisons in Life

This particular pattern begins by actually referring to itself as a language pattern. This in itself helps to dissociate the listener. By starting in a rather odd way with an announced hypnotic language pattern, or collection of words in this case, the client may assume a more detached position to consider these words, but then the language pattern ends up going into the very process that needs to be examined and seeks to alter the perspective of the listener.

This collection of words as you hear them is intended to convey the concept that all comparisons exist out of context. Most of us compare one thing or another to an item or items within a similar category. As a child, we may compare our height to a child to that of another child. We may compare school work or we may compare skills through competing to see who can run faster or throw a ball farther. I would suggest that we are taught to compete and that it is not something inherent in us. But regardless of this last idea, we start comparing early in childhood and tend to compare in age-relevant ways throughout our lifetimes. And the influence of early comparison results in a tendency to do what's known as a red herring search, finding what you already believe no matter how much contrary information you must ignore. You become convinced that you are destined to pull a particular card from a deck, the 10 of Hearts for example, and if you do not pull it as the very first card, you keep pulling out cards and ignoring them until you find the 10 of Hearts and then announce, "Aha! I knew it!" What do you know if you get to know the other cards you had said no to?

The problem with comparing personal skills, traits, or attributes is that this comparing misleads us into faulty conclusions begging for generalizations about self-worth. The process and principles of making comparisons involves first choosing a skill, trait, or attribute. This then severs off the chosen item from the whole of items existing. If we use the math skills of a fourth grader as the chosen item, we must first remove all other skills from view. The result is a time and space warp.

By a time and space warp I mean that we remove the history of math skills and we do not know or account for future math skills, a vertical plane. We also do a space warp in that we ignore all other current, horizontal, cognitive, and academic skills, let alone any other personal skills that coexist in the present. Therefore, it seems that all comparisons are misleading in that each is out of context. The most we can do is compare within our self, across time relative strengths or over time for personal progress. Now you can get on with what matters, choosing a task, a goal, identifying, finding, accessing, and using the resources you know you have.

White on White: Detecting Contrast

This story describes a process of developing the fine art of noticing differences between items in our world. The ability to notice differences provides a crucial and useful awareness. With this awareness we can treat each situation as the unique situation it is. We can also find more available choices and even choose our resource state better since we do not look for problems and react out of fear. Noticing differences in situations can permit us to gain freedom, rather than just repeating history. The pattern presented utilizes confusion to dissociate the listener, and then gradually introduces the general skill category of identifying differences. The client is then invited to apply this in her life.

Sometimes I play golf with a friend. Actually sometimes I play golf with several friends. Sometimes I play with two others so that three of us play and sometimes with three others and we make a foursome. For some reason four golfers in one group seems to be the ideal and maximum number. I don't know why, but then once I wonder why I start to ask all kinds of whys, you know? Like why in a car's automatic transmission is the gear for reverse in line before the one for drive? I don't know either.

Anyway, in this golf story, and you don't have to know anything about golf to understand this story, so don't worry, one of the guys who I play golf with has a serious eyesight problem. And at first that may seem odd, or even strange, but this guy has worked out a system where he can see enough to aim the ball in the general direction of the hole and then, knowing the distance, he can swing the right club. It is really very interesting to watch, and he can play pretty darn good golf, probably like the average golfer, but then you consider his handicap and it's really amazing.

The more I play with this guy, the more I learn about how his system works that lets him play so well. Not long ago we were playing and the golf course was in a sort of unusual condition. In the spring, just like folks do at their own home gardens, the golf course does some spring sprucing and amends soil and grasses. On the greens, where the hole is and golfers putt, this golf course had just been aerated, making these little holes all over the green and then they covered the green with a thin layer of sand. So, from a distance, the green was white.

Well, because we had never played when the greens were "white", I had never had a chance to see how he sees his golf ball when it is on the fairway or on the green. I knew he sometimes had some trouble finding where his golf ball was laying but I did not know how he actually went about spotting it. So this day with the "white" greens allowed me to be privy to another part of his system. And it made perfect sense once I heard it and thought about it. He finds his ball by noticing the contrast between the surface, the ground colors, and his white golf ball. From a distance, the contrast may not stand out so much, but once he gets closer, the contrast becomes stronger and more defined and then he notices it.

So with the "white" greens he really had to look very closely to find and notice the contrast between the much more subtle contrast of colors. It can lead to some very interesting observations about what we observe in our own surroundings and the contrasts that we notice from a distance and how these contrasts become this much easier to find when we look closer. And then I wonder, and you may wonder as well, just what you may find that you find contrast in and with…and how this contrasts with your old style of observing and what you find you observe you observe new…with this new style and how you can…and will benefit from this in so many ways as when you really think about it, there is contrast in everything, or else everything would really be all one thing or maybe no-thing so that you can find the unique something in everything this way now and how…you will…use this, maybe differently sometimes and the same sometimes and maybe again unique to each time because no two times are really the same, just like before and now are now different, aren't they?

Dogwood: Planning

This language pattern addresses foresight as an important factor in making effective life changes. A general broadening of awareness is encouraged by noting the various interacting variables and how a change in one leads a change in all. The overall goal is to activate use of foresight, patience, and flexibility.

In our backyard we have a dogwood tree. This tree sits on one level of our yard, while just a few feet away, the yard has another tier that is lower by about two feet. You could look at it the other way and stand below and notice that our yard has another tier that is raised about two feet. This dogwood tree is in good health and blooms beautifully in the spring. You know the white petals of a dogwood tree. At night when we look out over the yard from the second-storey window of our home, it looks like the dogwood tree is lit with the bright white petals standing out against an otherwise dark setting. Later in the spring, when the white petals fall off the tree, it looks like snow has fallen…but…you know how…to tell…the difference.

And while this dogwood tree is healthy and pretty to look at, we considered removing it so we could plant some other, more sun-loving plants in the space now made shady by the tree. And as we imagined removing the tree and then thinking about space left, we realized that all of the plants now existing underneath the tree are shade lovers. We have several types of ferns and other flowers that love the shade and thrive there. If we remove the dogwood tree we would then expose and harm the existing plants, creating a real problem where there is not one.

What thoughts move through your mind now as you think about your plans in light of what already exists, and how these changes may change what already exists, and if this will be best in the future you want?

Cues in Detecting Differences

This metaphor is designed to help the listener sort through an environment to become aware of differences. Differences exist between each existing people, places, and objects. Knowing how to discriminate between similar yet different circumstances can be very helpful. One of the key skills of people who function in healthy ways is an ability to recognize the difference between two or more conditions. Recognizing differences prevents generalizing, which permits more personal precision, flexibility, choice, and freedom. With such dynamics in mind, notice how this story leads the listener from a very common experience to then accessing skills that detect differences.

> When I was about five years old, my mother, father, and I would go to the grocery store. Back then I had little idea of what was in the grocery store, just that what my mother brought out in these brown paper bags we'd take home and eat. I had no idea that the store was organized with specific places for certain items for particular purposes. To me, from the outside and at my age, the grocery store was just a pile of food or a mass of groceries. What you wanted would surely be all in one place in there and you'd just go in and get it...as though they'd know what you'd want and just have it there for you.

> Well, when we went to the grocery store, my mother would go in the store and buy the groceries while my father and I would stay in the car. It took about 30 minutes for my mother to get the groceries or at least that what it seemed like. But you know we each have this interesting ability to lose track of time when we are doing something else and focusing carefully on it. And who knows just how children perceive time anyway? So to have something to do while we waited for some length of time we played a game. It was an interesting game to me and we could play it anywhere we waited. We would always park in the parking lot in a space that would allow us to look out at the main road in front of the store. And certainly back then I had no idea how you go about finding a parking place in a parking lot by looking at the cars already parked and then realizing that in order to find an available spot you'd have to look for where there was not a car, and pull in there.

> This game we played involved my father and I looking at each car that drove by and, as quickly as possible, we'd identify the kind of car it was. We would use categories like the brand names, Chevy, Ford, Buick, Oldsmobile, Pontiac, or Chrysler to identify the kind of car that was driving by us on the road. So the way to get good at this was to start looking for and noticing certain unique features common to the different brands of cars. Maybe it was the taillights or maybe it

was the bumper or fender, or the front grill or the roofline. But we'd sit there and carefully study each car for its unique features that related it to one of the brands. At first we'd have to look at almost the whole car to notice specific features that set it apart. This took a while to accomplish. Later, we were able to look at several features, maybe the taillights and front grill and the bumper and shape of the trunk, rather than the whole car. And then, the more we noticed, the more we were able to just look at one or two features, the shape of the hood or the shape of the front door, and know immediately, with great accuracy, the kind of car.

And you might find that you find you possess this ability to look at certain parts that let you know exactly what this part is of that you know and use to make better informed decisions with more accuracy and efficiency as you think about the past and ways you would have known, and then the present and the future knowing ways that you will have known you know now.

Falling to Stand Up: Juxtapositions to Increase Awareness

This language pattern relies heavily on confusion to shift the listener from all-or-nothing thinking to a more flexible continuum of thinking by broadening awareness. It seems is quite easy for each of us to do all-or-nothing thinking where we view life, self, or others in black and white terms. This is especially likely to happen when we experience strong emotions. But, as you know, we leave out the vast majority of information and experiences by thinking in this polarizing way. Sometimes by actually inviting thinking to the extreme, a person's thinking naturally begins to notice and fill in the great canyon between the two poles.

With the language pattern below, I aim to stretch polarity of thought even further toward the extremes to create a natural stretch, and then rely on a natural cognitive response of "snapping back" to grayer areas of thought. The principle at work here is that if you go to an extreme first, the listener will often react by naturally favoring a more moderate perspective. You might consider introducing this language pattern at either of two particular junctures.

The first would be right after the client has expressed some polarizing thought on an issue. Another opportunity may present itself after you summarize what you have noticed to be the client's polarizing thinking over a period of time while discussing a particular issue. You could introduce this latter observation by stating how you continue noticing a trend in the way the client perceives their situation.

> You know it occurs to me and maybe to you too, that certain things repeat themselves in this world. Some things just naturally occur over and over in some very predictable cycle. You can think about the seasons and find that summer follows spring and the spring follows winter and autumn follows summer. You can think about day and night and how day always follows night or is it that night follows day. It is sort of hard to know which came first and then which follows which but we do know that one comes after…zero. Unless you think about time and then one comes after twelve and that's odd even until you remember the countless uses for numbers. Just how many ways are numbers used? How many things do they measure and how many increments do they express? From light years to millimeters and beyond, in each direction, it stretches infinitely.

> And at the same time it is also nice to know that each spring we can count on the rain to help the growth of the grass, flowers, and crops. The rain falls so the plants can stand up. Which also reminds me of a client I spoke to in the past, which I guess is redundant, who said she could not stand to sit. And I thought how true this is because these are mutually exclusive. You really can't stand to sit or sit to stand, but you could stand after you sit, or vice-versa. Otherwise you remain standing. And yet this only accounts for a small portion of the distance between sitting and standing, because there are many points in between sitting and standing such as bending, both forward and backward, rising, turning, and various other postures, let alone various motions.

> And in this world, which is really only part of a universe, some places have a seasonal tradition where certain occurrences take place in certain seasons, when the swallows return to Capistrano the residents officially consider it summer. It's fascinating how these birds flock to this particular place, they are drawn magnetically it seems. My great…aunt told me of an experience that she had when she was living in California. She told me of how she learned to get rid of a fly that had flown into her house. She told me that, to get a fly to go where you want it to go, you have to go where you do not want it to go. You know, it's about gaps, filling and reactions.

And sometimes opposites attract, creating a wonderful blending of colors, shapes, and resources that blend into such beautiful useful ways. We may find that we like it so much that we look for how to use it, opportunities you know? And so you can scan your environment looking for and noticing left, right, and in between, for the many ways and opportunities that rest in between finding that you can also scan the environment within yourself and notice, finding the range of possibilities like shades of green, blue, or red and then the target and how your aim is true.

Horizon: Dealing with Ambiguity

The hypnotic pattern below addresses the inevitable presence of ambiguity in life. The language pattern starts by referencing a safe external world then utilizes confusion techniques to shift focus to the internal world within. The purpose of the pattern is to invite tolerance of ambiguity within oneself, as this invites patience and, ultimately, additional information about the self or a situation to present itself to us. If we strain and reach out for information or answers before the bigger picture becomes known, we may jump to conclusions or find we make choices based on very limited information. If we take too patient a position, on the other hand, we may find passivity leads to an equally poor method of gaining more insight into situations. The language used suggests we mix tolerance of ambiguity with a proactive approach designed to provide more factual information. A more informed position allows better decision making and thus, more effective results.

You know, when you think about it, the horizon determines just how much and how far you can see. If the horizon out in front of you is flat, you can see a lot of comings and goings. You can see things off to the left, not left off, and you can see things off to the right, maybe right off. You can see things close and far with ease, just depending on your vision and how clear the air is. But when faced with a rise in the horizon, some of your vision is lost. You can only see that which rises above the peak, giving you *only* a peek of what's going on, on the other side. Now taking a glimpse within yourself. What do you do with what you do not see, yet knowing it is there, here? Going by feel you get to see inside yourself and notice how you deal with what's missing. Do you tolerate the absence of information about what's over the hill, wait to find out later, after all, what's the danger? Do you fill in the missing pieces, missing the peace is within you? Do you, if it's important to you, move closer to get a better and bigger, more informative look and see?

Replacement Parts

This brief pattern aims at those people who tend to be overly critical and blame themselves for errors. The actual error, if there is one, stems from what we think, not from our self. The idea behind this language pattern is to depersonalize one's erroneous thinking to then draw from the well within to replace old, ineffective thinking and acts.

> You know replacement parts are made and so this presupposes both original parts and the need to replace them. If there were not parts or need to replace them, then no replacement parts would exist, just like erasers come attached to pencils. Of course, you do not replace what is not there nor has nothing wrong with it in the first place. Remember the old adage, "If it isn't broken, don't fix it"...unless it's fixing to break. And just as an aside, the term pre-supposing presupposes supposing, doesn't it? So what makes you think this change is not good? Maybe just this old thought is not good and needs to be replaced by a new thought.

Yellow: Expanding Perceptions

This simple pattern involves starting with a single pinpoint perception, then adding the emotions of a true story to provide emotional energy as fuel for change. The true story starts with awareness of just one shade of yellow as the metaphor for a single, all-or-nothing perception and the choice it creates. The language then progresses to help the listener expand their awareness, from one to many to all possibilities. A timeline is utilized within the language pattern. This is designed to help the client evolve beyond what may be the limited thinking held over from childhood to a more expansive, inclusive perceptual ability. Once the pattern is delivered, you can then ask the client to apply the expanded perception to whatever issue had led to the client feeling stuck.

> A friend of mine was telling me about how when she was younger and growing up at home, her mother was very particular. So particular that her mother would tell her what colors to wear and not to wear so it would look good with her skin tones. One such color she was told not to wear was yellow. I wondered aloud, just how many shades of yellow are there? She told me how back then there was really only one shade of yellow. I thought how interesting this was and began to move forward in time using my own memory to notice how she was right way back in time but then, as I moved forward in time I began to notice how some slight variations in yellow began appearing. Then as I continued moving forward in time using my memory, I noticed how several more shades of yellow appeared and soon there was an even broader range of yellow showing up over time. And as I continued moving forward in time, using my own memory, I noticed how these shades evolved over time. It then began making quite a spectrum of yellow from the lightest to the darkest and then mixing slight bits of other colors in with the yellow, so that it is still yellow yet, showing a different shade, tone or hue. And then after I began to notice and realize the wide range of yellows, I started thinking about other colors, watching them expand in each direction from the first one I knew on and on.

Things that Were but Are No Longer: Leaving the Past Behind

This language pattern is designed to help the client let go of old behaviors, emotions, beliefs, or memories so as no longer to be encumbered by negative, distracting aspects of life. The language attempts to re-categorize an old bit of information, belief, or response that still exerts a negative influence on the client. The old information shifts from active status to the category of things that were true, but are no longer true. The method is to help the client first clearly identify what they want to remove from active status. The client is then presented with a series of examples of truisms about things that were true but are no longer true so that they can re-categorize the old information. This is accomplished by the client associating the old memory or response with the truisms, thus placing the old within the category of things that used to exist but are no longer. For those who utilize NLP, this language pattern represents a linguistic version of the visual technique *mapping across*.

Some things do not go on forever, and it's better. You may have been in the fourth grade at one time and been there all school year. At times you were absent, though you always went back to fourth… until…you were no longer in the fourth grade even though the fourth grade continues existing, you are elsewhere and never went back, only forward. Some things were but are no longer, and it's better this way. You know everybody has a birthday but you only have one first and one second, then it's gone and one third and one fourth, one fifth and smaller as time goes by and you get bigger. You move on finding only what is ahead.

And as you look ahead you can notice how we all sometimes find our future to be clear at times and other times sort of foggy. Just like everybody has had the experience of driving in their car and maybe it was a wet day outside and your windshield fogs up, making it hard to see. Then you turn on the defroster, even though it's not really frost on the windshield, the warm air blowing from within warms and clears the windshield allowing you to see your way clear.

Maybe at some other times you've been driving in your town or a town you are familiar with and noticed an abandoned old building on an abandoned piece of property, you call an eyesore. Later you notice this building has been removed, a new one built to suit the tenant and the grounds nicely landscaped, improving the site. Some things are no longer, instead replaced and improved.

And while your conscious mind can't possibly come up with all the examples of things that were in your life and for the better, are no longer, your unconscious mind can quickly and easily sort and find the countless times when things were and then were not and it was faaarrr better…Though your conscious mind may try, it can instead just choose to relax and trust that your unconscious mind will find and remember all those times, finding comfort in the memory. In fact, the more your conscious mind relaxes and enjoys, the more your unconscious mind can find, feel, and enjoy the memories of things that are no longer yet better because, you know more after the change you find to be true. Your conscious mind can just sort of enjoy riding on the memories of your unconscious mind, or your conscious mind can just receive the pleasant feelings that your unconscious mind finds and sends or maybe your conscious mind can experience the comfort and enjoy pleasant feelings right along as your unconscious mind does the same. So you don't even know if you remember but...you do enjoy this most curiously pleasant experience right along, aren't you now? And it's always now you know.

And when something that was is no more and life's better for it, you may wonder if it will return. Sometimes people say things like "It will happen when you least expect it." But the word least is a comparative word, so to make the most accurate, all-inclusive comparison, you'll have to just go on forever feeling better to find out.

Or, if you stop expecting, going to a whole new way, then what had been your past expectations become irrelevant anyway. Just as there are car models that are no more, replaced by more effective, efficient vehicles that have new names and functions. And there are words that are no more because they have no application since what they represented no longer exists, replaced by a new item and a new word to go with it.

What's New: Acquiring and Using New Awareness

The language in this pattern is intended to expand the listener's awareness, adding new dimensions. Here I challenge possible ingrained tendencies that too quickly integrate new knowledge, rather than allow the new to provide more ongoing benefit. The intent is to prevent new knowledge from becoming too quickly incorporated into an old map, thus taking the edge off the new. When we discover something that adds to our awareness, we can maximize its benefit by letting it influence and reconfigure our old map for as long a possible.

There is a continuum in the integrative process as well. If we integrate the new too soon, it loses its novelty and potential to help us adjust for the better. If we leave the new out of our map for too long, we never integrate it and may not fully utilize it because we have yet to make sense of it. The inspiration for the language pattern that follows is an attempt to balance new information and, hence, increased awareness and ambiguity.

I ask this because I do not yet know, how long is something considered new? You know, when you first learn something and decide it is new, which comes from comparing the new with the old, and if differences are found, we think we have found something new that we had yet to know. And for how long do we consider this new? Maybe it depends on several things, and the least of which is time. You can think about things that you know now that were once new. And you can think about things you just learned, and then you can think about things you don't know yet, but will know in your future, going there these will be things you will know and beyond to these things you will have known. Then you can think about the ways that these things remain new by looking at the different dimensions of this new awareness, the different way of looking at the different ways of looking at...things and the many, many discoveries. So you can look at what you know that is new in many ways and then you can begin to think about the many applications of each of the many dimensions...giving you multiple dimensions and multiple applications. And, of course, in your future you can remember these learnings and notice how you keep them fresh and how you refresh them and even if they may not be new they can renew and you can re-use these...time and time again making many new things of this that you have yet to know but will.

Patterns: Similarities and Differences

The words in this pattern are intended to help the listener become more aware of tendencies and patterns within the environment and the self. This awareness can then be used to navigate more ably through various situations in life. If we can learn how to identify patterns of behavior or response patterns we can better manage certain predictable patterns life presents. How do we repeat patterns of thinking in the self? How do we repeat mood patterns or states within our self in response to or in anticipation of situations? And how do we display behavioral patterns through life? If we can identify our patterns or tendencies, then we can offer ourselves choices rather than repeating habitual patterns. We can also benefit by learning and knowing how to identify patterns in others so that again we can choose rather than blindly react.

Pattern, patterns. It's not really a pattern until it repeats. Some would say noticing something just one time is a novelty while noticing the same thing twice is a trend and after the third time it's a pattern. I don't know for sure but you will...come to notice patterns perhaps first by going into your past and maybe by noticing what you noticed last that you did not like and if it repeated itself before then. There might be a pattern of certain items that repeat that you notice and you know how to intervene like a switch changes the track of the train moving it differently. Or maybe you can and will notice patterns in yourself that you can notice when things went well for you and just what you did that you repeated to create a trend and even a pattern. Everybody has some success at some things and you can notice where you feel the best and notice that there is a sort of pattern to this process that results in success...that's right...just notice and highlight. Just like everybody has seen wallpaper that has a pattern on it. And you know that the wallpaper did not just unfold in one continuous sheet to cover the whole wall. The paper was applied in sections, being very careful to notice what the pattern is and where the pattern leaves off, there are certain cues you know, so that it can be picked up right there with the next section, continuing seamlessly, matching up to create one continuous look...at your success and the patterns you find you find that work so well for you. Where it starts, perhaps upstairs as you think in the attic of your mind, creating ideas and plans that you then bring outside to complete noticing the small pieces that let you know what the pattern is and how to continue it so well to complete success. And this smooth feeling because you know that when wallpaper is first placed on the wall there is a space of time that allows adjustment before it dries in place. Positioning carefully, lining it up, and then smoothing the bubbles away, what a finish. Then the next piece is moistened appropriately, placed, adjusted just right, and then matching the pattern well and smoothing the bubbles away to complete. Repeating this until the walls present this pattern arranged in just the right sequence to make for the look and feel you want. And you can think about the various ways and the various patterns and the various parts and skills that combine to make this so effective by noticing these patterns so that even before you start you can choose the pattern you most want to show and see...how you can choose just right for the time, place, and situation...the patterns of patterns and how they all fit together, creating so well.

Conscious–Unconscious Mind Split

This short section within the perception chapter includes uses of hypnotic language to emphasize the conscious–unconscious mind split. One way to think about human function and dysfunction is to look at the relationship between the conscious and unconscious mind. While there is controversy and diverse theories about these two forces in us, I believe that at some level the struggle within us for better functioning is a battle for supremacy between the conscious and unconscious mind. Our conscious mind seems poorly suited to run our lives, given that our conscious mind possesses limited awareness and information-processing ability. Yet, it seems our ego, sense of worth, or self-esteem, reside within the conscious mind. It seems then that we feel we must prove our worth over and over by "doing it myself", letting the conscious mind with its limits manage life.

This insistence on "doing it myself", letting the conscious mind manage life, may actually set us up for repeat performances of limited competence, thus continuing the need to prove competence over and over through the ego. With this concept in mind, finding ways to help a client shift from the conscious mind to the unconscious mind as a resource can greatly aid healthier functioning in life. If one views the unconscious mind as possessing a wealth of perhaps unlimited resources and awareness, then leaving life management to it may permit much more effective choices in life. The following brief collection of hypnotic language patterns attempts to demonstrate a shift from the limited conscious mind to the unlimited, resourceful unconscious mind in "solving" problems. In essence, the more you can help clients access and draw from their unconscious minds, the more effectively they will be able to live.

I used the following language pattern with an adolescent who called me from school on her mobile phone when she was in emotional distress.

I did not expect to resolve her deeper issues in this phone conversation, but did aim at settling her down by shifting her to a more comfortable, peaceful state of emotion. The path was to help her shift from her conscious mind to allowing her unconscious mind. This shift was designed to allow her to release the negative emotional and mental restrictions of her conscious mind.

I knew that Jennifer had been developing her spiritual self recently. One of the ways she had done this was to light a candle and then pray while looking at the candle flame. Jennifer had told me that this way of praying calmed her greatly and allowed her to overcome other life distractions during and for quite a while after praying. In the phone conversation with Jennifer, I first let her describe to me what was happening in the moment that upset her, what she felt and thought.

After she expressed herself, I said to Jennifer,

> Remember the setting you use in your bedroom to pray. Remember the way you light the candle and settle yourself into a comfortable position, the way you like, and begin watching the flickering flame. It moves from left to right, rises and shrinks and then rises again. The colors go from orange to blue to some reds and maybe even some white. And you can notice the how the flame encircles the wick and then up to the tip of the flame and how as you pray you find you feel closer to your God and safer. Think about and imagine a light so bright from this candle, knowing its true source that when you focus on it, it makes everything else invisible, you can see only this light, not anything else, only this light…And the feeling this allows as you go forward, illuminated…protected…guided by this safe, reassuring, loving light.

The remaining hypnotic language shorts are intended to play upon and accent the split between the conscious and unconscious mind. You may choose to incorporate them within larger hypnotic language patterns. You may also find them useful as strategic responses to client issues. These shorts may act as brief metaphors or scripts to invite exploration of client's unconscious material.

> A sign off in the near distance with writing on it that you can't quite make out. The curiosity drives you to look closer and you see. Then driving by next time, you know without seeing.

> You can stand for two hours or more at the same spot along a river and the scenery around you never changes, yet the water is never the same. And just watching the flow and observing just what is flowing as you remain standing still watching and seeing the changes as the water you now see is now past, and the new water you see is present, and then the next and the next as you just stand still as the water moves, flowing endlessly as you notice that not just you are not moving but you can also extend your awareness to notice the ground and how it remains still and just follow it as your eyes move across the still ground moving, moving toward the moving water

noticing how the ground remains still right up next to the edge of the water where you see stillness touched by moving, receiving the waters as they pass by contributing and depositing and removing, transforming the stillness through moving.

Thinking about your car or the vehicle you own, remember a time when you sat in the passenger seat for the first time when someone else drove. Remember when you sat in the back seat (or imagine this) of your car and notice what you notice from this new and very different point of view. Notice as you look up the ceiling of the interior and you can see things you had not seen before.

Everyone some time or another has taken a particular road on a familiar drive that they made over and over, many times over. And suddenly, one day, you notice a house or a building that you'd never seen before. You wonder if it's been there all along for these weeks, months, or years and then realize it must have been there all along because you just went by there the day before.

I saw an elderly woman crossing a busy road, walking across. And I wondered at first and was concerned as I thought this elderly woman might be in danger. But then I realized she was elderly and therefore was quite able or she would have died young.

And as you sit here…listening to my words, how do you know you are not at home? And how do you know you are not in your car? And yet…you can easily imagine yourself at home and I wonder just which room you are in. You could also imagine yourself in your car, perhaps driving or being driven, or even in the back seat. And maybe you've had the experience of standing in the front of an empty classroom and noticing the incredible view this affords as you can see the whole room and every desk within.

Have you ever noticed that when you're nearest the source of a noise that it interferes with you hearing what others say in the distance yet they, because they are removed, can hear you very well and then the principle involved?

A friend of mine was telling me about a cousin of his who told him about a very unusual [*or any descriptor*] incident. While my friend was talking to me about this experience I was really listening and wondering. And just then he said to me, "I see you hear I feel curious [*or any other state you want to plug in*] about this situation. In fact I am so curious that I feel drawn in to explore more and discover what is at the bottom of this so I can find out what went on before this happened and what other choices may exist."

Have you ever traveled to a new and different place? Maybe it was a different town or maybe a different state. You had directions to this new place but, since you'd never been there or made that trip before, you did not know quite where it was or just how long it would take to get there. Once you get to your destination and do what you went there for, you start making your way back home. Did you notice how it always seems to take much less time to get back home? Why, do you think?

Have you ever traveled out of town? Maybe you traveled to a different town or a different state. And when you got to this different town you noticed that it had a road of the same name as one back home. You may have felt surprised or maybe felt more at home though you knew you were not at home, different yet similar. And maybe you traveled to a different town or a different state that had a different area code. And when you looked in the phone book or saw advertising that listed phone numbers of local businesses they had the same prefix as phone number back home and you thought how odd even. You knew you were not at home but there was this similarity yet difference.

Your conscious mind can go right on sleeping while your unconscious mind arranges covers and shifts to find just the right position to sleep comfortably.

Did you notice when you were growing up that your yard, front, or back seemed so big? I mean it seemed really huge and almost endless, and maybe the same with your house. And have you ever revisited this same yard as an adult and notice just how small your yard and house seem now?

Chapter 6
Hypnotic Language Scripts Addressing Time

This chapter addresses the role of the concept of time in creating and solving personal problems. Each language pattern presented in this chapter utilizes time as its primary focus. As a concept, time has been invented by human beings and in part functions as a way of marking events relative to one another in a linear fashion. We compare the past and present and an imagined future. Life events are linked in time to form a sort of gestalt. This temporal gestalt contains emotions and beliefs associated with the event at a particular time. Problems or solutions tend to derive from a time-event-emotion-belief gestalt exerting a limiting or enhancing influence, respectively, on present and future.

Notice how time-oriented gestalts are stored as memories and then exert influence, since we tend to avoid cognitive dissonance. We seem to seek consistency in a rather automatic, habitual way unless we decide that the present and future exist independently from the past. More importantly, change can occur when we recognize that ingredients of time—events, emotions, and beliefs—exist independently rather than fused together in an inseparable gestalt.

Time tends to bind memories and events together. Yet time is always passing, eroding the past and present, leading us to a new and different future present, provided we decide to make different choices than we did in the past. Time is one variable that can be utilized to make change happen. Since time is the capsule wrapped around an event, using linear thinking, we may unwrap time and find a time-warp of sorts. By removing the time that binds, we can free the elements of past events to discover new and different meanings and associations, expanded awareness. Here is a selection of time-oriented hypnotic language patterns using the concept of time as the means of opening up and dismantling gestalts, restoring freedom of choice.

Past Reflections: Time-Related Beliefs

Here we examine how we may draw on our past to create negative beliefs about the self. We sometimes misunderstand past events, assigning errant or erroneous meanings to them. We also tend to freeze our beliefs, never updating them, yet drawing on them for life decisions in the present and for the future. This process is like keeping an old pair of shoes from when you were 10 years old and insisting that every new pair of shoes you buy must be this same size.

The therapeutic idea introduced in the following language pattern is that the past is just that—past. And the present is separate from this past, new and different. This difference requires a fresh look, updating by releasing the old, assessing and embracing new beliefs about self based on updated, current information. This particular hypnotic language pattern proceeds to induce confusion and disso-ciation from the past to examine old ways and then point out new ways of making sense of self and life.

Just recently I was reading a book. I was not at home but I'm not quite sure where it was that I was and read what I'm going to tell you. Do you ever remember things but you're not quite sure where it was that it happened? Maybe you can narrow it down but the exact place or time eludes you. Well, that's what I'm experiencing and I guess everybody experiences this some time or another. Of course, we don't quite remember when either.

Now, you know that almost everything you see is the result of light reflecting off it. Other than the sun, light bulbs and fireflies or lighten-ing bugs, and lightening, everything you see just reflects light. And the principle here...the further away from the object, the longer the delay in the reflected light getting to you. Now this light tells you what you see, once it gets into your eyes and your brain processes the information. At first, you might think of objects nearby and how short a time it is, given the speed of light, for you to see and identify the reflected light.

But the further away the object is from you, the more the delay in receiving the information. Now notice this principle holds for many areas, not just light. It's true for sound. If you ever notice some event you went to, to watch, maybe a sports event or maybe fireworks. If you were a good distance away from the site of the action, you can see before you can hear. You notice the action and then shortly thereafter, you hear the sound from it. And this is really something to behold since the sound actually happens first but the sight is first seen. You know, light travels faster than sound but the sound set the light in motion. This mismatch between sight and sound is different than the old movies you may have seen where the voice and mouth movements are out of synch. That's always kind of funny to see, you know where the actor's mouth moves and later you hear the words or first you hear the words and you know what the actor's going to say even before they say it? Doesn't that take the impact out of it?

Taking this reflected light idea a bit further, astronomers study the stars and the galaxy and the universe as far out there as they can see, knowing it goes beyond this. They use very powerful telescopes to look at distant stars. One thing they have come to learn is that the activity they observe when looking at a star is always several light years or many light years old. The star is so far away that it takes a long time for the light emitted to reach us.

The sunlight you see today, saw yesterday, or will see tomorrow is 8 minutes old. The sun sent this light out 8 minutes ago. It's old light and I doesn't mean a third less old. It is what the sun sent out 8 minutes ago and it just now reached us so it's not current, it's out of date. Who knows what's going on there right now? The principle is, the further away the object, the longer the light takes to reach us. And the light is always old or older. It's out of date and not current.

Now, looking into your past and remember everything you look at is reflecting old light, outdated and not current information. The sights and the sounds are no longer. It would be quite an error to look to your out-of-date, never updated past and reflect on it. It would also be an error to think your past reflects you when the present is really current always moving. Get out of the shadows cast from your past and bask in the new light you know of the present. Notice what's new and what you know, not k-n-e-w but k-n-o-w now different from then, separating. And what of the light reflected from your desired future? This is interesting and attracting. What does this illuminate for you to see and know, feeling, leading you to this future light that you desire? Going there now, noticing…realizing…feeling…and seeing how…you will…shine then and now illuminating various resources within….

Time Distortion: Outside Time

In the process of inducing a trance, it can be very helpful to distort time so the unconscious mind may better disconnect from old ways and become receptive to new ways. Distorting time can generally aid in inducing a trance as some of our old ways are time oriented. We learn how to activate old beliefs and behaviors morning, noon, or night. The more we separate time from various thoughts, emotions, and behaviors, the easier it is to shift into a trance state where we can access new ways by choice. In a general sense, a trance loosens old connections, encouraging disconnection and replacement. One way to loosen old connections is by distorting time.

Another benefit of distorting time is that this also seems to bring about dissociation. By losing track of time, we may also find we lose track of self, since time is one of our basic orienting modes. Thus, time distortion represents a general point of entry into trance and dissociation, enabling application of these methodologies to what had been a problem. The patterns below represent examples of time-distorting hypnotic language that may be used to bring about or deepen trance. These patterns can also be used to access the resource of time distortion so this can be applied to an area where it will bring benefit, such as losing the ability to mark time by using panic episodes.

What if you could not remember or lost all ability to know when it was that you had your last panic attack and thus not knowing when (time oriented) to experience your next one since you used to think it occurred in a time-oriented fashion? You would never again know when to have whatever it was you used to have according to the clock because you cannot time.

Below is a collection of time-distorting hypnotic language patterns.

> In most people and maybe in you as well, what seems to make for time passing faster is interest and eagerness, an enthusiasm that allows a person to truly immerse within an experience such that this is all they know like when you taste a certain food or that special dessert and the rest of the world disappears, you know the time. And the time when a movie is just so fascinating and the story is so good

that you lose yourself and all time as you just step into the story and experience it fully. So you can notice your eagerness and interest...in...feeling comfortable [*fill in state of choice*] and allow these feelings to sort through everything else and sift, tossing out or ignoring anything else while you eagerly sort with great interest, finding your comfort. While you find and keep your focus on your comfort your interest can grow as your comfort deepens and your comfort can deepen as your interest grows, wondering and noticing...more comfort...as you notice more comfort with deep felt eagerness and interest in feeling your comfort such that this is all you know now.

With or without words, we tend to explain events with material readily available, material just before and just after an event. This easily leads to faulty cause-and-effect logic. What other material before and after may have influenced the significant event? How do you know the material just before and just after actually had anything to do with the significant event? What material is not present that may have had an influence, frustrated needs on one or more person's parts? What did you not focus on just before and after the event that you feel sure had no influence on the event? How do you know this? How do you know the items you think influenced the event really did influence the event?

You can go into your future, well after you've solved this old problem to the place where you feel the great sense of achievement and accomplishment, resolving, settling in and enjoying the feat, well past the relief. And you can step into this wonderful place and you can notice a door that leads to your past, which used to be your present but from your future is your past. Knowing what you accomplished and the feelings this brings. You can identify the ingredients you used to achieve and inform your past you know. Or you can simply bring your future past you into your future present showing how and sharing how and knowing how with full support because it works for you now and then return to the present and begin again, yet differently now.

Past is Past: Present Solutions for the Future

This brief pattern is simply designed to address one's tendency to look to the past for solutions to the present. Not that past learning isn't valuable; it is vital. But sometimes we can fixate on the past and miss lessons available in the present, along with solutions such present learning may provide.

You know some counselors use what's called hypnotic language to help others make changes. It is an interesting process. I really enjoy speaking in hypnotic language and so I will...here and you may wonder if I've already started. But to find out if I have and just when, you'd have to go back into the past, searching for what appears to be the beginning. And then you'd miss that which is now the message and useful information for you. So you can now notice just how the past can interfere with what's important in the present and when you think about it, the only way we have any problems in the present is to think about the past in the present, superimposing the past on the present which is really a super imposition, when what we really need to know is...now available...which means you are past your past. And your present is...more important than your past because the present holds solutions which allow you to make your future present...what you want now, aren't you?

Past the Moment to the Future: Expanding Time Awareness

The language below is designed to help the listener disrupt the Gestalt habit of using proximity and consider a larger timeframe. The purpose of considering a larger timeframe is to allow clients a better sense of continuity and awareness of how the past fits into the present, creating the future. Through this time-orienting process, choice is emphasized as a conscious creative force in making the desired future come into being.

Sometimes we tend to try to explain certain events using just the information right there in the moment without a glance to the past or the future. While you may be able to do this tunnel vision trick, you may not be accurate. Sometimes we try to force fit information into a belief, or at least this is what I believe. And everybody has heard stories about someone who tried to fit themselves, feet or body into some piece of clothing because they need to make this the truth about themselves.

And you know that everyone shops at various stores for various things that they want or need. Maybe you've been shopping, maybe at a store that sells interesting decorative items and you saw an item that you just loved. But you did not know yet where this item would fit in your home or office. Even so, you felt so compelled to buy it that you did, realizing that you would find out sooner or later how this item will fit into your home or office, just right. And maybe at some time in your past you've found some unidentified piece or part on the floor or in your yard like a piece of something bigger. But you don't know what it goes to so you just keep it until you find where it fits, you know, consciously using your past now with an eye toward your future knowing you'll know it when you find it.

And then maybe you've had experiences, like everyone does sooner or later at some time where you make decisions in the moment based on some future plan. This way each decision you make in the moment collects, accumulating, moving you toward your future that you want, feeling very good about this decision. And yet if someone saw you while you were in any given moment gaining these parts that you assemble into your desired future it might not make sense to them but it does to you because you know what you want, what it needs and you know how to get it now...aren't you?

Before You Know It: Time Distortion

This script has many applications. You can use it as a means to activate time-distorting ability, then apply this loss of time orientation to a particular issue. You may also use this script and the time distortion it promotes to help a client achieve a better trance state and then proceed to multiple embedded metaphors with the goals of your choice.

It is interesting, what we each pay attention to each day. And you know we all pay attention to something all the time, whether we know it or not. Some people do what's called multi-tasking, paying attention to several things, alternating their attention between tasks. Some people pay attention to just one thing and go very deeply with it. And just think, while we pay attention to one thing all other things keep on going anyway, on their own, whether we pay attention or not.

And it's interesting how sometimes time seems to pass faster, even though time always travels at the same pace, your mind can alter the experience of time. Just like when you drive, especially when it's either repetitious scenery or familiar or both, while you travel at the same general speed during the time, it seems like you get where you are going in no time flat. It reminds me of a time when I was riding in the car my brother was driving through a neighborhood and said, "Does it seem like we are going really slow or is it just me?" I said, "I think we are all going at the same speed."

Sometimes while traveling you do not notice much and did not notice that you did not notice while focusing elsewhere. The next thing you know you reached your turn or exit and it seems like no time to you. You get there before you know it. But then in some ways you are always there before you know it because you first have to get there and then you can know it. And in a way you have to go there to know it but you're there before you know it. And sometimes people say that they look after themselves. But what about looking before yourself?

And the same thing can happen when you read an interesting, intriguing book or article. Maybe the words on the page occupy your mind or maybe your mind thinks of new thoughts while you read and then you go off in thought, and maybe you've often thought of losing all track of time. Your unconscious mind has some awareness of the material and some awareness of time while your conscious mind knows it just wants to think about these interesting ideas and how to use them. Or maybe your conscious mind considers the details of how to use them, while your unconscious mind begins enjoying them right away, as it knows how and then shares with your conscious mind. And either way, whatever way, you can lose track of time so easily that you can't even remember when that you find what you want to find and use it before you know it.

And this reminds me of a story about a heating and air conditioning repair guy who made a house call to work on a heating system that had stopped working. In just a few minutes the repairman emerged from under the house and presented a bill to the homeowner. It was for $300. The owner was upset and asked why the bill was so high for such a short period of time. The repairman answered that the part was $10.00. The other charge was for knowing what was wrong and how to fix it so quickly. And you can think about the know-how and fix how now…repairing and restoring to full use and more.

Things That Do Not Last: Reframing the Past

The purpose of this script is to assist the listener to reframe old information. The intent is to reduce or eliminate the influence of old memories by re-assigning them to the category of things that do not last. You need to consider the client and whether or not they have suffered any recent significant losses or deaths of loved ones. If that is the case, I would suggest you not use this script. The process in the script below involves first accessing some event that the client may wish to render dormant with its associated emotions. Once the event and its influence have been identified, you may then help the client into a trance and present this story. The client can then consider how life experiences include many transitory elements. After sufficient examples of such, the client will have opened up this cognitive file and may then place the problem memory within it.

Some things do not go on forever, and it's better. You may have been in the fourth grade at one time and been there all school year. At times you were absent, though you always went back to fourth... until...you were no longer in the fourth grade even though the fourth grade continues existing you are elsewhere and never went back, only forward. Some things were but are no longer, and it's better this way. You know everybody has a birthday but you only have one first and one second, then it's gone and one third and one fourth, one fifth and smaller as time goes by. You move on finding only what is ahead.

And as you look ahead you can notice how we all sometimes find our future to be clear at times and at other times sort of foggy. Just like everybody has had the experience of driving in their car and maybe it was a wet day outside and your windshield fogs up, making it hard to see. Then you turn on the defroster, even though it's not really frost on the windshield, the warm air blowing from within, warms and clears the windshield allowing you to see your way clear.

Maybe at some other times you've been driving in your town or a town you are familiar with and noticed an abandoned old building on a vacant piece of property, you call an eyesore. Later you notice this building has been removed, a new one built to suit the tenant, and the grounds nicely landscaped, improving the site. Some things are no longer, instead replaced and improved. The clothes that you outgrew, the clothes that did not hold together and were replaced, the whole category of products known as non-durable goods, they are here for awhile but do not last and are not meant to.

And while your conscious mind can't possibly come up with all the examples of things that were in your life and for the better are no longer, your unconscious mind can quickly and easily sort and find

147

the countless times when things were then were not, and it was faaarrr better. Though your conscious mind may try, it can instead just choose to relax and trust that your unconscious mind will find and remember all those times finding comfort in the memory. In fact the more your conscious mind relaxes and enjoys, the more your unconscious mind can find, feel and enjoy the memories of things that are no longer yet better because, you know more after the change you find to be true. Your conscious mind can just sort of enjoy riding on the memories of your unconscious mind, or your conscious mind can just receive the pleasant feelings that your unconscious mind finds and sends, or maybe your conscious mind can experience the comfort and enjoy the pleasant feelings right along as your unconscious mind does the same. So you don't even know if you remember but you do, enjoy this most curiously pleasant experience right along, don't you now? And it's always...now you know.

And when something that was is no more and it's better for it, you may wonder if it will return. Sometimes people say things like, "It will happen when you least expect it." But the word "least" is a comparative word so you'll have to just go on forever to find out. Or, if you stop expecting, going a whole new way, then what had been your past expectations become irrelevant now anyway.

Because it's all about evolving and improving and refining so that what was becomes better, turning into what is and paving the way for what will be better. Just like there are automobiles, cars that used to be produced but are not longer being made. There was the model A which is named appropriately but there is yet to be a model Z but there are Z cars around. Maybe you have seen Z cars. There are other cars that are no longer made for many reasons, different reasons but always good reasons so that the cars now are better and the cars to come will be even better, looking back than to find that there will be even better than what was before that is no longer and not even knowing any more, just focusing on what is and will be now and in the future which serves you better.

Utilizing the Now

The purpose of this language pattern is to address and prevent regret over lost opportunities in the past. It seems we each possess a tendency to focus, however briefly, on some lost opportunity in the past. If we let go of past disappointments and hurts we can more successfully satisfy needs in the present. A past disappointment or felt loss might revolve around relations with parents, children, adult relationships, our work, or some other facet of daily life. The goal of the language pattern is to assist the client in letting go of past losses, an oxymoron of sorts, since you let go of what is not there. Abandonment of the past allows a client to pursue what is desired in the present or future.

> It seems that people experiencing emotional distress often endow the past with a one and only opportunity to satisfy a particular need. The person may take a specific and narrow focus on the past event. In other words, the person may have wanted to experience love from a parent. This love would have supposedly led to higher self-esteem and a better sense of self-worth. Believing the parent to be the only source of this love and, therefore, the only source of satisfying self-worth, bad relations with this parent doom any opportunity to experience improved self-worth. But a more accurate and beneficial interpretation of this supposed lost opportunity comes with both a different time orientation as well as a more general perspective. Living in the past prevents awareness and more self-worth in this case. From the specific situation, we can find numerous ways to satisfy this need. The need is general and a source is specific. When emotions run high we often have a hard time separating the two. Once we separate the general need from the specific source we become free to find a better source, ultimately self or beyond.

In the language pattern that follows, notice that the time is reoriented in a fairly specific manner. The available opportunities to satisfy needs in the present and the ultimate self-directed effort toward these needs get worked in after the appropriate time orientation is gained.

> Just recently, I was playing a game of pinball and I learned something. You know the game: there's a small silver ball, some flippers that you operate and you make points by hitting targets. The ball bounces all around the board, off the walls and the bumpers and various targets. Once you set the ball in motion by deploying it, every position of the ball is the cumulative result of every other preceding position of the ball. This might be a bit confusing since we tend to think that what we see in any given moment as the result of what we saw *just* before. And while that's true, this is true of what we saw before and before and before that, all the way back to the beginning, which then accumulates through time into the present, contributed to by *every* preceding second first.

So, while I was playing, I was trying to maneuver the ball to hit certain targets. Sometimes I had good results and sometimes I did not. Each game only gives you a certain number of pinballs to use so you try to make the most of them. I was doing pretty well with the first pinball and then all of a sudden the ball went out of play and I lost it. My first thought was about the lost opportunity and how things were working well and then *gone*. Then I started to feel regret, sort of leaving me in the past trying to revive what was but is no longer.

And then this thought came to me that was unexpected. I thought I was just playing pinball and not really engaged in any thought beyond right then and there. I had this thought; it was odd even. There is nothing in your past that your present cannot provide. I disengaged from the past and what's unavailable and immediately launched the next ball, knowing the opportunity available now, the only one which can accomplish what I want anyway, until the next and then the next in the future which will then be the present opportunity available holding all that I want again. So I quickly contained myself after visiting the past and disengaging, then visiting the future and disengaging, knowing I will be in my future present later and just devoted myself to the current present...opportunities that hold all the things that allow satisfying goals now.

How satisfying to know that you are competent enough to be competent because of course you achieve when you use what you already possess within and then all this implies about you and you can only achieve what you are capable of. And you know, sometimes people use the phrase over-achiever. But this is really an "under-expecter". Trees can't be over-tall, rain can't be over-wet, flowers can't over-bloom and the sky can't be over-blue, just over you and you are as capable as you are and no less, only more because each of your achievements rises from multiple abilities always being added to...unlimited. It's just a matter of finding and using them and there is no limit to this.

Chapter 7
Hypnotic Language Scripts Addressing Behavior

The hypnotic language patterns within this chapter focus on addressing and altering behavior. Several elements such as perception, beliefs, and time orientation are drawn upon in the process. But the aim of these patterns is to effect behavioral change in line with the client's desired outcome.

Beach Trip: Weight Loss

The following scripts were used in working with a woman who came to me wanting to lose weight. Brenda is a woman in her mid-thirties. She was about 50 pounds overweight according to her estimate. Brenda lives alone and works as a school teacher. She not only teaches school but also involves herself extensively in several after-hours school-related activities. In addition to this, Brenda assumes a caretaking role with her somewhat disabled father, who lives on his own. Over time the situation in her family has evolved so that Brenda is also the sole food provider for her father and sister, who each live on their own. Her sister comes to Brenda's home, usually in the early evening to pick up food and then returns home. Brenda then takes the food she prepares for her father to him.

Brenda's daily schedule includes coming home from her teaching and extracurricular activities about five or six in the evening. Brenda then starts cooking large quantities of food for her family, sampling too much as she cooks. She then delivers the food to her father, and sometimes to her sister, returning home to clean up her kitchen and finishing by about nine o'clock. Brenda describes experiencing much frustration over this arrangement with her family, yet feels obligated to continue this arrangement.

In a slightly larger circle of her social life, Brenda appears to be someone who invites others to turn to her for help and sustenance in different ways. Her students, her fellow teachers, and her family all feed off Brenda. Placing herself at the center of numerous people's lives has created quite a problem for Brenda, yet this also meets many needs of hers as well. I did not feel it was my place to work toward unraveling Brenda's entire life structure, as her current life structure played such a vital role in providing her self-esteem. I determined that Brenda would not be willing or open to such a drastic change. Instead I focused on how to maintain the general structure Brenda needed, and at the same time incorporate flexibility, balance, and increased self-protection, establishing boundaries to prevent her overextending herself. I also sought to activate foresight in planning so that she would rearrange some items to better organize her daily schedule.

The metaphor I chose to describe to Brenda is based on my knowing that she enjoys traveling and that she also invests time and energy in her pre-travel routine, ensuring safe travel She had told me that she greatly enjoyed going to the beach, and so I used a trip to the beach as the metaphor through which to deliver multiple healthy messages.

Choose a method that will allow you to help the client achieve a moderate trance level and then relate the following narrative.

> As you enjoy experiencing this deep feeling of relaxation and the calmness that accompanies, I want to tell you a brief story. This story is about two good friends. These two friends decide to take a trip to the beach. They both enjoy a good road trip, especially to the beach. And the day before the trip they decide what they want to take with them. This includes a variety of things, some they know they will use and some they bring just in case. They also know that if they really need to, they can buy something there. So they plan and pack carefully, leaving some room for future interests they may have down the road.
>
> The next morning, the driver carefully inspects the vehicle because you know how important this is. She looks at the tires and checks for their proper inflation, that they are neither over- nor under-inflated, examines the tread and takes stock of the other important ingredients that will make for the safest travel. Now they begin their traveling trip, and she knows that at some point along the way they'll get

off the main road for one reason or another. And she also remembers that, if for some reason she takes the wrong exit or turns the wrong way, she can instantly correct this by turning around and getting back on the right road. She knows that while she may be tempted to feel temporarily frustrated and or even disappointed, as soon as she gets back on the right road, immediately they will resume moving toward their destination and feel good about this.

Now they return to the road and making fine progress, they arrive at the beach. Instantly they take in the sights and sounds they so enjoy. During their stay there, a brief shower comes along. Now, they were prepared and had brought an umbrella. But this umbrella was not quite right for the situation. They could hold it to one side and one of them would be completely dry while the other would be half wet. They could hold it to the other side and one would be fully dry and the other half wet, or they could hold it in the middle and they'd each be half wet. So they decided to buy a new umbrella that keeps them both dry.

Later, after the rain stopped and the weather became clear, she takes a walk along the shore line, you know, walking so that the breaking waves just come up and over her feet, and then returning back. She could look higher up the beach and see by the still wet sand that the tide had been higher but now the tide was going back out moving toward low tide. As she continued walking, enjoying the sights, sounds, smells, and light breeze, she noticed something interesting when she looked down at the waves coming over her feet and returning to the ocean. When the water moved back out to the ocean, the flow would make them sort of lean toward the ocean, almost feeling pulled toward the water. It was sort of dizzying. Then she found that if she fixed her eyes on an object in the distance, she could walk straight. She noticed a pier off in the distance and she looked at it, which was quite interesting actually, and she found that could walk straighter and handle the current better. She continued walking and enjoying, also realizing that she would soon need to return home, taking with her the wonderful memories collected.

On the return trip they move on down the road and she discovers that the car needs gas. So she finds a gas station and stops there to fill up. Now she's gotten to be quite an expert at filling up. You know how the gas filling the tank makes a particular sound and as the tank gets fuller the sound changes. She has learned to listen for this sound of being nearly full, recognizes this, and stops short. This way she keeps from overflowing and spilling gas on herself, smelling it for hours afterward.

Returning to the road, it felt much quicker on the way back, you know how when you're going somewhere new, it can feel slow but the familiar return seems to come much faster. And as she drove to her town and saw the familiar sights and landmarks, she turned toward her neighborhood. And everybody's had the experience of traveling on a familiar route and then suddenly noticing something new yet it must have been there for a long time. Well, she noticed what looked like a new tree in a neighbor's yard. She saw an oak tree. But it was really well developed and so she knew it must have been growing there for some time in a healthy way. She also knew that its roots go as deeply into the ground as its tallest branches go high, a most secure arrangement.

She then noticed there seemed to be a ring of space around certain other trees, no grass or flowers were growing in about a 3-foot ring around these certain trees. Then she remembered how some trees secrete an herbicide of sorts that prevents anything else from growing in a small ring right around them to keep away competition for the nutrition, allowing the healthiest growth and development. And as she continued making her way home and inside, she noticed her familiar surroundings, knowing that she's home, feeling good, just enjoying these feelings as they are absorbed and also generated from within. And you can now begin noticing the surroundings here as you come back to this room, feeling good.

Behaving with Foresight

This language pattern was used in assisting a client with weight loss. While the pattern utilizes perception, I placed it within this behavior chapter since the goal of the pattern is to change behavior. But this pattern, with its emphasis on foresight, can apply to many different issues. I think of foresight as being one of the three primary cognitive resources that helps the client find solutions. In addition to foresight, patience and flexibility bring much needed ability to solution finding. When thinking about a client's presented problem, in some ways one or each of these three cognitive skills is missing from the problem-making process. By injecting and activating these three skills, solutions often come into the client's awareness.

You can think about and remember times when you may have thought ahead. And, of course, you use your head when you think ahead. And maybe you think back to when you thought ahead and find that you found good reason to think ahead. You know, you wanted to prevent or create something that was very important to you so you anticipated the way things would go depending on the choices you made. And you then decided to make the choices that would make things go your way.

Everybody has had the experience of planning to go outdoors and take a look at the weather to decide if they would need an umbrella, you know, you consult the forecast. Maybe you look at the TV or listen to the radio, tuning in the channel you know will tell you what you need to know about the future. Or maybe you just take a look outside and look up at the sky and see the clouds. If they look a certain way, you figure it will rain.

And then if you find that it is expected to rain, you take an umbrella with you. You do this because you can look ahead in time, sort of time travel to the future and notice what will and what will not happen if you have an umbrella. And since you don't like the picture, feeling, and consequences of getting soaked, you take an umbrella with you to shield you from the unwanted rain. Because you know the feeling, you get soaked and you can't see so well and your clothes get to feeling very heavy and you can't move very well and even your shoes feel heavy. And instead, when you have this umbrella with you, it is interesting and maybe even feels quite secure and reassuring when you take that umbrella with you. All the while you know you have the instant ability to protect and prevent what you don't want to happen, feeling better instead.

And certainly everybody has had the experience of planning to take a vacation. You might remember times when you traveled and you knew where you were going and could really anticipate being there with great excitement. You would think about the number of days you would be there and think about and plan what to take and where to go. There are many things to take into account when planning and this ability to anticipate, use your knowledge and this thing called foresight. You know foresight is this ability we each have that lets us think about the future while we are in the present, knowing now what will happen then if we do certain things. We can see, hear and feel the future and make decisions now that will fit well with our desired future. And when we use this foresight well we find we make choices based on what we want our future to be like, so that we like our future, what a fine fit this makes.

And everybody has heard the phrase "four eyes". Sometimes people who wear glasses are called four eyes. And while this is not foresight, you could think of your conscious mind as having one set of eyes and your unconscious mind having another so in a new and different way, you could have four eyes, giving you "four-sight". Your conscious mind can see what is around you while your unconscious mind can see how your current choices will turn out into your future, knowing now what you want then to happen now. And what needs to happen now to make then what you want. Your foresight can enable you to look at the present and know what certain choices will look like on your future. So this allows you to choose easily and enjoy the power of knowing you choose well.

So you can think about this foresight and this ability you have to anticipate, you know look ahead. And maybe you can anticipate your foresight or maybe gain foresight as you're anticipating your future, just right. And sometimes you find that your unconscious mind uses its foresight to anticipate and choose accordingly. And sometimes you find that your unconscious mind anticipates your foresight, making choices so easily and quickly.

Maybe your conscious mind can just be informed of the results of your anticipating your foresight and maybe your unconscious mind can just enjoy knowing it knows what's ahead, already. Then your conscious mind can easily find this is true. And I wonder if you find that your foresight increases the more you use it or if your anticipating ability grows faster now. And just how far into the future should one look is good to think about. You can think about how far you need to look to look how you want to look, knowing what to say "yes" to and what to say "no" to.

Some people might consider anticipating and foresight to be like a flashlight. This beam can shine from you for you telling you what's in the present and how choices will show up in the future. This beam from the present into the future can reveal how your current choices will play out in the future and what effect they will have so you can know if you should or should not. And as you think about this shining beam from your present into your future you can also get a glimpse of how you want to look and will appear. As you notice choices leading to this and your feelings about these choices and the results and how others respond so well. Absorb this and fill up on this feeling fulfilled. So you get to not take in some things but to fill up on others.

Now notice this skillful ability to see your present and future with this light you now use. Notice how days of this skill lead to weeks of this skill. You know how some people after a good week say they had a strong week, they went a week strong. And this leads to months and years and even more of the feelings you want to have and hold within.

Then and now you can begin anticipating using foresight in a whole new way, seeing yourself as you like. You can use your foresight to anticipate this new way. You can see and feel this difference and the wonderful, satisfying feeling this contains for you, finding that this feeling is within you and remains as a result of these choices. With each of these choices, these healthy choices you get immediate gratification, knowing and feeling you chose the right way and the immediate benefits. And just how you will feel when you will have made these choices time after time, gaining the reward immediately leading to such a wonderful fulfilling feeling. Just notice this collection of choices out into your future. Your choice points you in the right direction, guiding you to where and how…you want to look as you look at this new look you achieve.

Barking up a Tree: Accessing Well-Being

The language in the pattern below is designed to motivate the listener to access greater well-being and make healthy choices in the present and in the future. It starts with some deliberate confusion in order to clear the way for deeper exploration of the unconscious mind's resources. This exploring is aimed at accessing awareness of good health in mental and well as physical forms. The listener can relate to the content of the story and apply it to self more easily by citing naturally occurring forms of how the unconscious mind looks out for one's best interest. Relating to the information and examples then serves to help the listener associate this new awareness of good health into his unencumbered unconscious mind to let it guide him to greater well-being.

You know, you can hear a dog's bark and you can see a tree's bark. Maybe the bark is off in the distance and maybe the tree is very close, noticing the variations of the bark. And then you can think about the trees that you are barking up and notice if they hold what you want. And maybe to get a closer look you can climb up this tree to find...that you can get a better view off in the distance, seeing paths, some familiar and some new, to where you want to go. You may wonder how you will know and it is really very simple because your unconscious mind is always thinking. You know everybody some time or another has what seems like ideas coming to them out of the blue, but really your unconscious mind has been thinking all along. It's just new...to your conscious mind.

You know...your unconscious mind is always awake, even when your conscious mind is sleeping. You may go to sleep in one position and...wake up in another. Your unconscious mind knows when to pull up the covers or push them down, depending on what tempera- ture you want to feel. Your unconscious mind moves you and turns you while your conscious mind sleeps and knows just when and how to turn you so you can feel more comfortable for your best rest. Meaning that your unconscious mind can remove the covers...from your conscious mind...revealing....

So you can turn your conscious mind over to your unconscious mind knowing that it knows when and how to move you to the most com- fortable position for the rest...of your life as you find you can move more comfortably this way from this point forward just trusting the moves your unconscious mind informs your conscious mind to make for your well-being now as well as in the future. Thinking and feeling about this well-being may allow you to notice all the ways you can find and feel this. You may notice how the more you choose this well- being the more well-being you experience or maybe you will find that your choices simply lead you to find and experience more well-being that naturally leads you to more, the more of these choices you make the more well-being. And you can notice well out into your future how these choices accumulate and the benefits that are in keeping...with your goals and purposes allowing you to this much better...achieve these and how this feels.

Back Up to Move Forward: Self-Support

This pattern aims to help a client access their internal resources and draw on internal self-directing processes. The idea for this pattern came from a discussion I heard between two people in my office corridor. The Ericksonian principle of utilization is put to work here to hear someone talk about backing oneself up. (The speaker down the hall intended the words in a different context of external backup, but I decided to take this backup notion and apply it to a strictly internal process.) I explored the idea of backing up in various contexts and meanings, then wove it into a hypnotic language pattern that hopefully will connect clients with their deeper resources. We should recognize that sometimes we do need to back up and start again, reworking some things in life differently.

> You know, we have many ways of moving forward, and sometimes things move forward while we stay still, giving the impression we are getting left behind. Just like you can stand at the side of a river, the river bank, and watch the water flow by and all the while you never move while the water never stops moving. And sometimes we move backwards, giving the impression that other things are moving forward or vice-versa. Most people have had the experience of being in their car, waiting at a red light with another car beside them. This other car began to move slightly backward and you, in your car began to feel as though you were moving forward, pushing that much harder on the brake only to find you were still and they were moving and then...orientation.

> But you know there are also many reasons why we don't move forward. One of them is a lack of trust in ourselves. You can think of self-trust as sort of engaging in a gear within that allows you to move forward. Or you can think of self-trust as a force that resides behind you, providing a push to you at just the right times in just the ways that you need. Or you can think of trust as being like an escalator, moving you up and forward while you just let it propel you. This strength beneath you or behind you activates when you trust yourself and accelerates in relation to your trust of yourself, supporting and moving you. Without this trust, you may feel stuck but you have only to trust in yourself and your knowledge of how to do to begin moving forward in just the right way at just the right pace.

> And you can think of self-trust that resides as this power right behind you, moving you as need be, as a form of backing yourself up, you know. So really you need to back yourself up in order to move forward, aren't you, now? You are not here because you are not able, you are here because you are and you know this deep within and more as it rises to your surface, moving you forward, your unconscious mind like a transmission getting your conscious mind in gear and the positive traction...results from all these things that are already deep within you.

Extra Special: Behaving Naturally

This story is designed to address the tendency in some people to try too hard to perform something in which they already possess competence. When I speak of performance, I am referring to anything from social interaction to musical or athletic performance or any performance utilizing a skill. If we just focus on what we are doing and allowing our ability to express itself, we will perform at our best. If we take a perspective that is external or extraneous to our skill or resource by wondering how we will perform or how others will perceive our performance, we diminish our ability. Likewise, if we doubt our ability, we may press or force our performance, interfering with our natural skill. This story reminds the listener that skill is sufficient to itself and needs only to express itself naturally.

Just about everybody enjoys going out to eat at a restaurant. You know, thinking about what to eat and where to eat, maybe remembering what you had there before or what your taste buds tell you they crave. And maybe you have a favorite restaurant or maybe you know someone who has a favorite restaurant. I'll tell you about an experience that I had recently at a particular restaurant. My wife and I went out of town, to one of our favorite places to visit. We really enjoy being there. This town is at the beach and we stayed at a place right on the beach. We could see the ocean waves and hear the waves. It was great and so peaceful and relaxing. We just started feeling more mellow from the first sight and sound of the beach and the ocean. We watched the slow rhythm of the water in the ocean. You know, it seems the waves move quickly toward the shore at first and then sort of fold over and get smoother and slower, gradually sliding up the beach to a brief stop and then slide back into the ocean. Amidst a most relaxing experience.

Once we got the ocean in our blood and thoroughly relaxed, we started getting hungry and we knew just where we wanted to eat. We also knew what we wanted to eat. We have a favorite restaurant in this town and so we headed there. We have been going to this same restaurant several times a year for several years. I guess that's several squared. It is a really stable establishment and so we see the same waiters there each time. And we actually had the same waiter several times and then began to request a table served by that waiter because he was so good. You know a good waiter is one who gets the order right and can anticipate needs and then meet them.

The hostess welcomed us at the door as we entered the restaurant on this day. We noticed that our favorite waiter was at work and so we asked the hostess to seat us at a table that he would serve. He came over and we exchanged greetings as he remembered us, and we told him how we had asked for a table he waited on and he was quite flattered. We shared with him how we knew what we wanted to eat and how we order this same thing every time we eat there because it is so very good. And it is really a one-of-a-kind dish.

The waiter took our order and then told the chef. The waiter also told the chef how we liked the restaurant so much and how we made a point of eating there each time we came to town. The waiter also told the chef how we ordered the same item each time because it was so good. The chef appreciates how we appreciate the food there. He decided to do something extra special for us this time. This particular dish has a particular sauce on it. So the chef put extra sauce on the food. But the extra sauce disturbs the balance of the flavors that makes this dish so special. The chef gives it to the waiter who then brings it to the table. We immediately recognize the excess sauce and move it off to the side, restoring the delicate, tasteful balance and then enjoy the meal as much as ever.

We then express great appreciation to the waiter and ask that he pass this to the chef. We follow this by asking the waiter to tell the chef, please don't do anything extra to this dish. It is already just right.

Four Seasons: Initiating Action

The purpose of this pattern is to address some superficial and deeper factors involved in time management and one's chosen pace in life. The first part of the pattern is designed to induce some confusion, thereby aiding trance development. The metaphor of the master clock and trying to keep up with it when the master clock is malfunctioning follows. The aim of this is to not only increase awareness of managing time, but also to encourage looking within oneself at details below the surface to seek a natural pace that is neither too fast nor too slow. Unpleasant emotional states are identified in the hypnotic pattern and relied on to provide the energy, which may then be used to motivate change.

Each of us seems to possess a pace matched to our own nature and lifestyle. The problem presented within this metaphor stems from dealing with surface details and micro-managing life, while the solution arises from examining deeper levels that exert more influence on life. The moral of the language pattern is to look within at deeper levels of self, finding and honoring one's true nature in a more synchronized manner that will lead to more peace of mind and better functioning.

You know, in some states here in the United States residents adjust the clocks according to the seasons. Most states use standard time during the shorter days of the year. But when the daylight lasts longer, people in most states change the clocks. It's not that you get more daylight but it's to stretch the daylight out another hour in the latter part of the day, just shifting the light to when and where it may be more useful. It's called daylight saving time, you know, you save it and use it later. I think a couple of states do not use daylight saving time, not that they lose any daylight by actual clock time, it's just that the light starts earlier in the day there. It's interesting how time just goes on but does not really care when it is, it just rides above, or meta, to real life which goes on anyway.

The available light at any time of the year varies according to the four seasons. You know, spring, up to summer, better than others and just fall into place, which is second to the winner. And when you think about time and the seasons you may notice that the measurements go from smaller, seconds first to minutes and then hours. Your next time period is a day followed by a week, though it may be a strong week and then a month and a year and…you get the pattern, smaller parts that make up bigger parts that make up even bigger parts that we call time. And we made time in a neat order, a predictable order. And you may now notice other neat patterns in your life exist in a certain order that you use in a sequence. But it is important to notice if the sequence is right or out of order, not working.

Many factors can influence things that malfunction out of order. If you change time zones but forget to re-set your watch, you're either ahead or behind. Sometimes the watch battery needs to be changed for a new, fresh one, or you may have seen these watches and clocks that have a mechanism for adjusting the speed of the clock hands. You can just adjust the setting to how you need to keep up with the right time, knowing what time it really is to do what you need to do, aren't you, now…Noticing…how much control this mechanism of setting the speed of the hands allows, you remember a story about a person who took a commuter train to work each day.

This train left precisely at 8 am, no earlier, no later, you'd think they could make up their minds. This commuter would pay such careful attention to the time and would carefully set his watch by checking one of those time services you can call on the phone. He got to the train station only to find the train had already left. He scrambled to find an alternative way to get to work and just barely made it on time. The next day he set his watch a few minutes ahead so as to make it to the train on time. When he got there the next morning, he saw the train in the distance, making its way to the city. So the next day, more determined than ever, he set his watch way ahead and carefully arrived even earlier than he felt he needed to. Well, when he got to the station, he saw the train pull away. Now he was really frustrated and looked at his watch finding that he was still early according to his watch. So he went to the station master and saw this huge clock residing just above the station master's window for all the commuters to see. He approached the station master and pointed out the difference between the huge clock and his own watch. After much dialogue and negotiating, the commuter and the station master took a look at the clock and then looked at the device that determines how the clock is to run, noting there is a dial to determine the pace of the clock. How interesting. This dial was set to the fast side of center and so gained a couple of minutes each day. It was noticed and easily agreed to set the hand of the clock back to a more consistent and regular pace so as to neither lose nor gain… time…is right as you set it so…. Now you know you can.

Just Starting: Maintaining Momentum

This language pattern is designed to help maintain momentum through process of change, sustaining change into the future. Sometimes when we start something we may fear it will end before we want it to. Then we may say to ourselves, "I was just starting to…" You can fill in the blank that follows with words such as "understand", "succeed", or some term suggesting improved performance over time.

The following pattern plays on this "I was just starting to…" senti-ment *before* a process or at its very *beginning* in order to help perpetuate the change initiated. Several benefits are intended. First, maintain the change so it becomes permanent. Second, a degree of natural concern that a newly implemented style may fade or vanish is addressed. A third benefit is more indirect. The listener receives subtle suggestions to continue deepening and expanding the new personal style. Deepening and expanding will enhance the quantity and quality of changes over time, refining and adding additional dimensions to a new style. So this language pattern begins with a general introduction, then expands into deeper and broader aspects, becoming an example of the concept it presents.

> Change can be very interesting. You know, it sort of depends what kind of change and in what way and when, timing you know. And change can sure be brief or it can be enduring, really forever, at which point in the future, it is not change, just permanent. And it seems the more important to us the more we may find we wonder if…it will last forever, making it permanent. Which reminds me of a sort of similar principle of how people sometimes save things, maybe some valuable item, waiting until they *really*, *really* need it, for the very most important time. Maybe it is a set of valuable china saved for a special occasion. Or maybe it is the last of a remedy for an ailment being saved for the most crucial time, the worst episode. I wonder, and you may wonder as well, how will you know until the whole of all time is at the end, since the most or the worst is a comparative. You'd have to wait until the end to know when the most or worst was and then it would already be in the past. So some processes last forever because of their purpose.

> Now sometimes people decide and design things that they want to use forever, not hold back, rather use fully and freely. And if this design to be used freely and fully is important it becomes valuable and some might wonder if it will first last. And if they indulge their fear they may imagine losing this new way and returning to an old way. And with regret they may imagine saying to themselves, "Oh, I was just starting to understand how to do such and such and was getting to be pretty good at it."

> Well, in another way, we are each just starting to understand many things and yet this understanding simply continues as you come to understand your understanding deeper, allows you to perform this much better. And with each understanding you can understand more deeply…you find that this ability just continues to go deeper and you can understand how to use this understanding in just the very ways that you understand knowing that you understand. You are always

and continually just starting to understand more because your understanding of understanding just goes deeper and better… all ways…you use it…and how exciting the present and future feel and become, the eagerness to understand more and what this brings, to you.

Plowing to Perfection: Action beyond Planning

The following language pattern addresses the tendency in some people to plan some action extensively without ever moving beyond the planning stage. Sometimes in the effort to plan an event to perfection, the planner gets bogged down at the planning stage. The metaphor presented below purposely describes excessive planning efforts made by an individual and then leaves the outcome open-ended. Over describing the planning stage stirs frustration in the listener, which may become useful energy available for change. Leaving the outcome of the story open-ended invites the listener to comply with the desire for closure. The drive toward closure can convert the raw energy stimulated from frustration into action toward a goal.

This story takes place out in the country, away from the city. And yes, you could say that "out in the country" already tells you it is away from the city because they are mutually exclusive. But some things can be mixed like a city in the middle of the country or a bit of country in the middle of the city. One of one does not mean none of the other. So out in the country there is this farmer. He has a large plot of land and has neighboring farmers on each side of his property. He enjoys good relations with his neighbors and they each share a common cause, pursuing a common goal so they feel a bit like they are in this together.

Well, this particular year, as with each year, winter gave way to a warming trend and this signaled that it was time to prepare the soil for planting. This farmer stood in his doorway and looked out over his acres. He knew it would be a pain to plow his acres but at the same time it was a source of pride for him, and he began imagining just how he'd plow this year. He thought and thought. He envisioned this and that and various ways to design his fields to maximize his yield.

He developed a plan and got up early one morning to start the process of preparing the fields. He hopped on his tractor and fired it up. The rumble of the engine fired him up and boy was he ready and motivated. He could feel the surge of energy as he imagined plowing the fields into a thing of farming beauty. He took comfort and joy in riding along his open fields knowing that soon he'd see sprouts of green and then bigger and better. He also found it pleasing that he could see that his neighbors were also out and plowing their fields. From a distance he could see clouds of dust in motion surrounding his fellow farmers as they plowed.

He went this way and that way with blades gleaming, making sure and clear pathways for future seedlings. He spent several days at this task, not minding a bit as he knew he was making a path for nature to take its course. Once completed, he stood back and admired his work. As he surveyed his fields, he gradually started feeling twinges of doubt. Doubt gave way to uncertainty and then feelings of disappointment followed. Now he was dissatisfied with his plowing job. A deep dissatisfaction kept him busy most of the night as he wondered how to make things right.

The next morning he got up even earlier and started on his tractor. He would re-plow one section of his field. This would set things right, he thought. Once finished, he surveyed the field again. It did look somewhat better but now the other fields he'd plowed look somehow off. This day was gone and he'd start fresh the next day. He began at sunrise, making neat and clean rows, just so. In the distance he could still see a couple of his neighbors, dust clouds surrounded tractors plowing away, giving him some sense of comfort. But at the end of the day, he still wasn't satisfied with his rows. It just did not look or feel right. Again the next day he was up and at 'em. He plowed with vigor, trying to catch up to his neighbors. He knew they had finished as there was no sight or sound from the neighboring fields.

Once again, his rows, his fields did not look or feel right. He wondered and planned most of the night, rising the next morning to once again fix things to his liking. He fussed and tensed and gritted his teeth, trying to find just the right combination to make his fields the way he wanted. Finally he finished for the day and took a look. But again, frustrating, very frustrating to see, his fields were not done the way he'd wanted. So much time had gone by with nothing to show for it. He knew he had to get these fields plowed properly but couldn't seem to find the combination that satisfied. Now, in the morning, after this much time, he stepped out of his doorway and was stunned: an emerging carpet of light green could be seen on each of his neighbors' fields.

Memories: Behavior over Time

Here the listener is taken back into his past to examine previous choices. The purpose it to examine and break up old patterns that tend to repeat themselves out of habit. The metaphor of paved roads and the process of paving is used to describe perceptions of choice superimposed on an otherwise choice-filled environment. We tend to think our choices exist separate from the total of all choices, thus form limiting beliefs about self and life. This language pattern attempts to expand perception and, in so doing, to remove old paths and allow new routes to be traveled in the direction of choice.

Memories, past events making up the pavement that lays behind you through an otherwise non-descript landscape. It is these memories and the path they pave that seem to make you feel obligated to stay on the same old road, you know, just a pattern that repeats, repeats itself just because that's the way it was. The more you look behind yourself into your past, the more you lay your present path squarely in line with your past. It just seems natural to do it this way, without question. Yet, if you cannot, and will never travel over that same path in your past, what use is served by keeping this memory lane? And further, what was this non-descript landscape like before you traveled through it?

You have superimposed the events of your past over the infinite landscape. You then take the path as being real when it really is what is not real. It is not that these past events did not happen. They exist as real events. The problem is taking them as the *only possible* real events, thus confining yourself to take the consequences of these events personally and then form beliefs about yourself accordingly. Just because you have chosen particular responses does not make you anything less than every possibility. You are not the sum of your choices but your current life is.

The only real thing is the *total* landscape. The problem comes when you take your past as real rather than the partial truth that it is. A "problem" is not an event on your path, past, present, or future. Rather, a "problem" comes from a decision before any event, taking the path and events on it as actual and true. Problems stem from decisions that precede the identified problem. The identified problem is just the consequence of the problematic decision with a limiting belief (another decision) underneath this decision.

Have you ever noticed all the layers that go into making a road and how the pavement is just the culmination of all these layers? And when an old road is being taken up, you can see how the workers just strip away one layer at a time, removing the old road totally. And when you watch a new road being created, you can see the steps and layers that go in to this road, clearing and leveling the ground, then placing a foundation, later followed by another layer on this that is thicker and of more substance, only followed by another thicker layer of even more substance, sort of like how you go from a general goal to then add the specifics and then more specifics as you implement to achievement.

We just ride along the surface; what exists underneath provides the foundation. The surface cannot exist without the necessary foundation. All things were and always will be possible. Your choices are from the infinite array of choices. Selecting one does not remove all the others, they continue existing, what freedom. The structure of the universe does not change; you just choose a path within it to get you where you want to…go as all things remain available…always. This remains especially true for the past, the present, and the future.

Eat One and You Can Two: Modifying Impulses

This story is designed to address impulsive tendencies. The story may be useful for those who overeat but is geared more generally for management of impulsive behavior. Dynamics and concepts presented here may be used for those clients who need to learn ways to pace themselves rather than going at full tilt through a complete task. The first part of the story focuses on over-indulgence and eagerness, while the second part suggests alternative responses.

This story is for fun in your conscious mind and for taking in and digesting in your unconscious mind. The setting for this story is in a region of the world where rich farmland exists. The soil is so fertile that you can just toss out seeds and they grow magnificently. Now in this particular case, there are two farmers, a husband and his wife, who farm together and they love tomatoes. They absolutely adore red, ripe, juicy tomatoes. Well, they got wind of a special treatment that can be applied to the soil while growing tomatoes that generates the largest tomatoes you've ever seen.

Armed with this information, the husband and wife carefully set out just three tomato plants; yes, just three. And these three tomato plants generate only one tomato each. You see, the additive for the soil is so powerful that the tomatoes grow nearly as large as your head. The additive also speeds up the growth process so that the tomatoes are ripe and ready for the picking in just one week, seven days! Well, these tomatoes just shot up. On the first day the tomatoes were planted they were just small, frail looking plants with a few green sprigs.

The farmers went to sleep the first night and when they awoke and checked on the tomatoes, the plants had doubled in size and already had blooms. On the second night they went to sleep, woke up the next morning and rushed out to check on the tomatoes. Astonishing! The tomato plants had doubled in size again. This time they had green tomatoes on them the size of golf balls. From the very first night when this couple went to sleep they'd think about how the tomatoes were growing so much and could hardly wait to see the tomatoes in the morning.

They went to sleep the third night and woke up early the next day. They immediately walked outside and looked at their tomatoes. Absolutely amazing! These tomatoes were now beginning to get a bit yellow and orange colored, you know the way they get as they move toward red and ripe. They were now the size of baseballs. Each of the next two nights the farmers slept and dreamed about what awaited them in the morning. They'd go outside first thing in the morning and find that the tomatoes were getting huge.

By the sixth night the tomatoes were growing bright red and were the size of softballs. That last night they could barely sleep. Up before the dawn, they hurried outside. They grabbed a flashlight on the way out so they could see, one that had a strong, well-focused beam. They shined the flashlight in front of them, carefully choosing their path as they made their way toward the tomatoes. Suddenly, they both froze in their tracks. They could hardly believe their eyes and wondered if it was some sort of trick of light. Right there before their eyes were the three biggest tomatoes they had ever seen, bigger than they had ever imagined. Three tomatoes way bigger than their heads stared back at them; huge, bright red tomatoes. Each would take over a week to eat! What would they do to keep the other two preserved while they indulged in the one? Well they came up with a fine idea, you eat one and you can two.

Shoe Fly: Making Change

This language pattern addresses a common tendency to hold onto old behavior patterns long after they have outlived their usefulness. Sometimes what looks like resistance on the part of the client is actually hesitation. The client may hesitate to let go of an old behavioral pattern because he doesn't yet know what new one to adopt. Often we believe that the devil we know is better than the devil we don't know. The following language pattern addresses the dilemma of hanging onto dysfunctional old behavior instead of changing our behavior.

Not long ago there was a woman who was still wearing some old shoes that she owned. These shoes were from years ago and were quite worn. She wore them everywhere she went. But because they were so old and worn, they no longer fit her well and felt very uncomfortable. But she had no other shoes and just kept wearing these and trying her best to get around in them. Since they hurt her so much, she really limited her walking. She could only go a short distance before she had to stop. And the whole time her feet really hurt. As she strode forward, landing her foot on the ground with her worn shoes, her heel would take the full brunt of the concrete making for quite an ache. And as she continued moving forward she would feel the harsh, hard concrete on the bottom of her foot and then her toes would be forced to feel the unyielding concrete as she pushed forward, wincing all the way and dreading the next step.

While she struggled to walk and was restricted, she noticed how much more easily others moved about and she felt angry and jealous toward them. So every time she walked, she hurt inside and out. How much longer could this go on with no solution in sight? She dreaded her own painful walk and resented seeing others glide along so easily. At the same time, she knew she had to wear some shoes. These were all she had and the alternative was to go barefoot. This she knew she could not do. So on she went, feeling stuck with two undesirable choices.

One day while walking, she had to pause, as usual, before she could continue. In disgust, she looked down at the ground. Well, this was new. She looked at her own shoes on her feet and then looked at another pair of shoes on another person nearby. She compared piece for piece and found hers were different in just about every way. She noticed the shade differences, the soul, the heel, and the upper part of the shoes. She'd never noticed this before.

And then she wondered, were there others in addition to this? She began curiously and eagerly looking at every person's shoes. All the different shades, styles, and looks. The possibilities nearly over-whelmed her but then she realized…choices existed. She had not noticed the other styles before and now she did. She even asked several people where they got their shoes. They told her of various stores and she knew what she wanted to do now.

She made her way to the nearest shoe store and went inside. Here she noticed countless variations in shoes. She felt herself fill with excitement as she took in all the different styles. And this lead her to think about different situations and needs in her life, matching the style with the occasion, finding the best fit for her. She bought several pairs and knew now where she could find others if she needed.

She then took her new shoes home and went into her room, finding the best place to place her new shoes. She arranged them in a nicely visible manner so she could pick and choose for each day and for each situation, just the right pair. At times she would just look at her collection with great satisfaction and a sense of reassurance. She also knew that at times she would add to her collection of styles when needed. And she remembered what the sales person told her. There were new shoe styles coming out all the time. And there were even some styles yet to be developed, just in the creative stages now. And this really got her to thinking about possibilities.

With this in mind she felt eager to try on her new styles and go for walks, in great comfort as she easily moved about. She looked forward to this and enjoyed every step of the process from choosing the style, to putting them on, to wearing them in public as she walked as much as she wanted wherever she chose. She found that with comfort she could go to new places. She could walk further than she'd gone before, discovering many new things, creating many new ideas that only inspired her this much more. She now enjoyed the process, the discoveries and looked forward to remembering what she learned and the next new discovery.

Paper Airplanes: Matching Resources to the Situation

This story concerns matching and mismatching resources with circumstances to create the best outcome. Sometimes people choose the wrong resource or the wrong behavior in a given situation. Sometimes they feel compelled to force fit some resource or behavior to a situation. Such force fitting can stem from a need to prove competence or disprove felt incompetence. But unless the match between resource, behavior, and situation is a good one, a feared outcome may result. This feared outcome only deepens limiting beliefs the individual holds about himself. In this story, the theme concerns not forming limiting beliefs from misleading situations and outcomes taken out of context. An open-minded flexibility that allows better outcomes is suggested.

A few weeks ago, I was looking out the front window of my house and noticed my neighbor's grandchild in the front yard. He was standing out there with a sheet of paper, studying this sheet of paper very intently. He began to fold it and then fold it again in various angles. All this while a light rain fell. But you know children, oblivious to such a minor interference. His determination way outweighed the dampening rain. All the while he continued ever so carefully to fold this sheet of paper. Well the rain picked up in intensity and really began to come down heavily. Undaunted, this boy continued on his task. It became apparent he was making a paper airplane.

Once he finished the careful and precise folding of the paper, his initial flight was ready to go. He coiled his arm back and heaved that paper airplane as hard as he could at just the right angle to give it flight. But all it did was instantly fly straight down to the ground. Determined, he picked the paper airplane right back up and threw it again. The same results. Anger and discouragement showed on his face now. Quickly, he grabbed up the plane and threw again but with less conviction, almost like he already knew what would happen.

And it did. Now he just stood there, confused and frustrated. He did not know what to do at this point.

By now the rain was pouring down and the water was beginning to make a small stream along the side of the road at curb by his yard. Dejected he walked his paper airplane over to the curb and placed it on the stream of water just to get rid of his failure. He looked in stunned amazement. His paper airplane was now a most effective boat. It glided quickly and easily down the stream. How exciting! He watched with growing pride and satisfaction as the now, paper boat continued on its path. He followed it for awhile as it continued downstream, floating along with ease, just moving with the current. Now content, he went back inside to dry off and bask in his success.

It was then, in a moment of thinking, reveling in his success actually, that he realized, once the rain stopped he could make a flight-worthy paper airplane. Sure enough, once the rain stopped, he went back outside with paper in hand. He folded the paper in just the right way at just the right angles. Now he reared back and threw his plane. It glided along, so easily and freely, just as he planned. This was a lesson worth remembering. His sense of satisfaction and competence soared.

Pavlov's Cat: Learning through Anticipation

The following story addresses the process involved in lifelong learning. We usually learn in small steps that accumulate into larger scale learning. The metaphor in the story is intended to identify steps involved in learning and also the cues that allow us to combine new with old lessons, making for what might be termed complex learning. Identifying patterns that repeat and using this knowledge to skip unnecessary, obvious givens can promote faster learning. Underlying the metaphor of learning is the message of trusting others and, more importantly, the self.

Not long ago, my wife and I went to our favorite town for a long weekend. We really like this place because it is a nice-sized coastal city and also has islands just off the coast. We like to stay on the island so we can enjoy the best of both worlds, the beach and the city life. We rented a small condo at the beach and we had a ground-floor unit that was right on the beach. We could walk out of the screened porch and down the steps to the sand dunes and then across them to the water. It is really nice to see and hear the waves while sitting on the beach. And we could also see and hear the waves very easily from our screened porch. It is so relaxing and soothing. You know how your whole insides seem to slow down when you see and hear the rhythm of the ocean, just wave after wave, each more relaxing. You just slow to this natural pace that is so very comfortable and it lets you feel like you're floating.

We sat on the porch for a while during this sunny day and just watched and listened. We decided it would also be nice to eat our lunch out there on the porch. We prepared our food and brought it outside. There was a table out there along with the chairs so we had all we needed. We began eating and then, as minds tend to do when you really enjoy something, we wondered what it would be like to live there. We also wondered just how long we could keep this memory and the feeling with it in us as we went through our daily lives, sort of *it* living with *us*.

As we sat there on the porch, enjoying the food and the sights and sounds, we began to think back to another time on another porch eating another meal, this one at home. While we sat relaxing we thought about how one day at our home while we were sitting out on the porch eating lunch, a cat wandered into our yard. This cat slowly crept up toward us, no doubt smelling the food. But you could tell it was scared and nervous. We did our best to encourage it to come closer but it froze in its tracks. I decided to see if I could approach the cat but as soon as I made my first steps toward it, the cat bolted off to a safe distance, then turned and looked back at us. We had not seen this cat before and did not know if it was someone's pet or a stray.

The cat looked healthy. It had a shiny coat of fur and seemed well nourished. The coat was an interesting mixture of brown, black, orange, and tan in swirls of color. It was not a kitten and yet seemed still young. While the cat looked back at us, I tried to take a few slow steps toward him or her, but with each step the cat hissed with all its might and retreated. So I stopped and went back to the porch to sit and just watch. It seemed the cat did the same. At this point I decided that I could toss some tidbits of food in the cat's direction and it could eat them if it wanted. As soon as the food landed, the cat went over, sniffed, and immediately ate the food. I tossed a few more pieces one at a time and each time, the cat quickly ate the food. Soon we were through with lunch and so was the cat. We went on about exploring the town that afternoon.

The next morning, when I looked out through the glass back door to the porch. Who was there but the tabby cat, waiting for food. I opened the back door, which has a distinctive creaking sound when it opens. This time the cat seemed a bit less timid and backed up just a little rather than taking off so far. I decided that I would again fix a small serving of food, some leftovers we had, and I put them on a small plate. I put the plate out back at the edge of the porch and walked away to give the cat room to approach and eat. It was interesting to observe how the cat came up to the plate, sniffed and took one piece of food and then ran a safe distance away to eat it. Once finished, the cat came back and repeated this process until the plate was empty.

Even though the food was gone the cat continued to hang around, this time a bit closer to the porch. It seemed more comfortable. I just sat down on the porch and hoped it would approach. The cat sort of watched and stayed nearby but never came within petting range.

Later in the day, I got some dinner leftovers and put them on a plate. I opened the creaking door and put these on the porch for the cat, who was now staying closer and had not left our yard. As soon as I came out with the plate of food, the cat approached. This creaking door had quickly become a cue for the cat the food was in the offing. I had not even put the food down when the cat was at my feet, eager to eat. I put the plate down and stepped back to give the cat room to feel safe to eat. It seemed I became invisible once the plate of food touched down. The cat ate and this time did not haul each piece off to preserve it. Soon I became almost as leery of the cat as the cat had been of me, not sure what it would do if I reached down to pet it. So I just held out my hand, keeping it still and the cat thoroughly sniffed it. I left it at that for the time being.

The next morning I went to the back door, looked out and opened it with the familiar creak and saw this cat now waiting for me. It did not jump or seem edgy, rather calmer and more at ease. With no food in hand I reached out and let it sniff. The cat sniffed carefully and I could clearly hear it purring. After a couple of minutes I sat down on the porch and this cat came over to explore the porch and then just sat on the porch. I could still hear the purring.

After a few minutes I decided I'd fix the cat some breakfast and so I went in, fixed a bit of food while the cat looked in through the glass door. I returned to the porch through the creaking door. The cat was right there waiting for the food. I put down the plate of food and it ate, more slowly this time and not all at once, like before. I sat out there with this cat while and after it ate. I held out my hand and it came over, rubbing its face across my hand. As it passed I petted it along its back, which seemed quite acceptable. Now, as I went inside, the cat followed and seemed to want to come inside. But I did not let it in since this seemed a big leap. A moment after I got in I looked back out the door and there sat the cat as though it really wanted to come in. So I went back out through the creaking door and was greeted by an increasingly friendly cat, purring and allowing me to pet it. Now I was becoming more relaxed, catching up to the cat who seemed quite at ease.

Now that we were each relaxed and at ease, I let her in the house. She slinked in, sniffing and scanning yet still purring. She inched her way along the floor, checking things out and integrating her new environment. She seemed quite pleased and continued purring and exploring. To make her more at home I prepared some food and drink for her to enjoy. She did and seemed to relax this much more. This process of exploring and integrating her new environment continued until she'd explored the whole house. Although a bit cautious and slightly on guard, maybe more tuned in than anything, she gradually became quite used to what would become her new home. Now 8 years later she's still here and freely enjoying it.

As I was sitting on the screened porch, back at the ocean thinking, I was thinking back to the back porch at home and thinking how interesting it was the way this cat learned to anticipate things based on certain cues. She would pay careful attention to the circumstances, knowing what she needed. She would assess whether or not there was the potential to meet these needs and then determine if these needs could be met safely. She then would use this experience to adjust, making things easier for herself. After this worked, she would carefully assess her *next* method. Once meeting her needs this time she would then simplify the process and add some more complex needs to the situation to meet these needs. How fascinating to observe.

Once meeting these slightly more complex needs, she would simplify, using a more direct approach to meeting these and then even more complex, deeper needs. She did all this by watching for cues, patterns, and sequences of events to learn what leads to what starting in the present and moving forward, then looking in the past to review the effectiveness, only to move forward again, adding more simplicity, directness and so meeting deeper needs. And it's a good thing to get familiar with and meet your needs, simply...deeply... effectively feeling this now.

Save It All: Breaking a Habit

This language pattern addresses behavioral habits, presenting a story that may assist in breaking certain habits. The theme is habits that involve unnecessary use of resources or unnecessary actions. Positive emotions are tied to the new behavior that changes patterns. The metaphor of gum chewing is used to represent those habits that really get us nowhere, such as chewing gum and then spitting it out. The gist of the solution is simply to experience the reward associated with the behavior opposite that of the old habit.

There once was a man, or was it a woman? Well, I don't remember for sure but the point of the story is how this person decided to preserve something of great value. Of all things, this story revolves around gum, chewing gum, or bubble gum, to be more precise. This woman who loved chewing gum and blowing bubbles had a particular kind and flavor of gum that she enjoyed using to make her bubbles. It was a special flavor that really she liked, no regular gum for her. She liked peppermint flavor for many reasons. And this certain kind of gum blew just the best bubbles, really big and the gum's flavor lasted a long time.

She always made sure she bought several packs at a time when she'd buy the gum. And she always made sure she had several pieces of gum with her at all times so she could chew and make bubbles anytime she wanted. She had certain times she liked to do this more than other times but anytime was really the right time. Well, one day she had intended to have a piece of gum during a break that she knew was coming up soon. She took her break and got distracted and forgot to chew her bubble gum. At first she felt disappointed and then she began to smile. She realized that she still had this piece of gum available for her to chew whenever she wanted. She'd saved a piece, leaving her that much more.

When the next opportunity to chew her gum came along, she started to reach for that piece of gum she'd saved and then stopped herself. She thought about how earlier she'd saved this piece, giving her just that much more. A secret sense of pride filled her. She then decided to save this piece again so she would still have this amount of gum. The next time she bought more gum she began to really feel quite pleased with herself and the amount of gum she'd accumulated. This again left her that much more that she could chew.

Later that day she decided again to not chew this prized gum and instead save it so she could accumulate more. She went to the store and bought more gum and saved it as well. Now she really had a stockpile of gum and could treasure this. She never chewed gum again.

That's Your Job: Becoming Self-Directed

The language pattern that follows is about taking initiative in spite of others and their attempted influence. This pattern also contains elements that address intra-psychic dynamics to overcome auto-cratic treatment of the self. In the early part of this pattern, some confusion is used, relying on gestalt similarities; later the focus is self-directed behavior. Humor is also used, serving to disarm the conscious mind, thus facilitating the message's passage to the unconscious mind.

The metaphor starts out in what might be considered a relatively dissociated position for the unconscious mind, the listener walking within a department store seeking direction. The listener takes the role of dissociated from the larger self or department store. The story then shifts to what might be considered a more associated position for the unconscious mind, focusing on an employee of the department store. The ensuing conflict may represent a struggle between a self-critical, demanding stance toward the self and a healthy, self-fulfilling one.

> This is a story about a woman who worked in a shoe store, or maybe it was the shoe department of a large department store, you know the kind of stores that have several stories and each storey has several departments and, of course, each department has several stories of its own. But that's another story. You walk through the front doors and find the store directory, checking to find where you will find what you are looking for and make your way there passing by all kinds of different merchandise, from different states and different countries, nearby and far away and while curious you, you leave them to get what you came for.
>
> One woman, an employee in this department store, worked in shoes. And this is not like the old joke about the man who worked in

women's shoes. She worked in and wore shoes at the same time. One day she had a customer, a very demanding customer. This customer came to her and wanted to try on a particular pair of shoes. Once the saleswoman found and brought the shoes to her, the customer sat in a chair while the saleswoman sat across from her on those funny looking stools. You know the ones with the small padded triangular seat and this sloping, ridged black surface for the customer's foot. The customer put her foot on the black platform and just sat there. Each waited for the other and then the saleswoman asked the customer, "Aren't you going to try on these shoes?" The customer replied, "That's your job."

So the saleswoman tried the shoes on herself, walked around, and said, "I'll take them." She rang up her own sale, getting a nice employee discount, thanked the customer and went on about her business. Now, this is turning the tables on someone, finding the pivot point, the fork in the road, knowing when to pick it up and when to put it down, walking in what seems like someone else's shoes only to find out what you want and what fits, feeling so good that you have found your path that leads to where you want to go, and you just can't wait to get there.

The Bridge: Weight Loss

The following language pattern concerns weight loss and leaving past ways behind. This pattern uses the metaphor of a bridge to represent change, then moves into an embedded language pattern about fine-tuning one's lifestyle. The metaphor of tuning in a radio station to gain balance and clarity is used to convey this message. It also suggests accessing states and behavior that bring further positive change.

And as you make your way onto the bridge, that piece that helps you reach the other side…get to where you want to go….notice where you came from and the ways that formed you…and now where you are going in a new way. Allow yourself to continue crossing this bridge to where you want to be. As you make your way down to the other side you may do like other people: turn left right after the bridge or maybe turn right having left your past behind to move forward….

And this process reminds me of a song I heard recently on the radio. You know, the new radios have a digital tuner that displays the frequency. But the older radios had a tuner knob that you'd just turn either direction to get a station. These tuners you turned until you tuned into the station that you wanted, turning that dial until the sound went from static to clear. And then, almost by necessity, you'd turn the dial a bit more just in case somehow the sound came in clearer. But it only got more fuzzy and so you turned it back the other way until you could clearly hear the station you wanted to hear, the one that played the kind of music you like, the kind that you feel inside, that gives you joy and energy, making you feel good, making you want to move. Wait no more is the name of that song. And it got me to thinking and maybe it will get you to thinking as well about...since you'll get where you want to go sooner or later, later or sooner, why wait, just do it now, you know, so you will...have and do what and where you want...aren't you?

Day Begins Before You Awaken: Time to Change

This rather unusual pattern relies heavily on confusion and time disorientation only to bring the listener back to the present with a different perspective. The purpose of the language is to help the client expand and shift their concept of time. This conceptual shift then permits more flexibility of thinking and the breaking of old habits, replacing them with new, more effective ways of behaving. As the therapist, you may find this pattern can be used to open up a client's awareness in general, making for better assessment and change of specific personal styles. You can elaborate on the language pattern to include issues tailored to an individual client or just apply the new awareness to old styles to amend them in a conscious manner.

You know, it usually seems and it may actually be true that your day starts when you awaken. But it also seems true and may actually be true that the day starts before you awaken. And then you are faced with the growing question of just which day and which night and when it starts and when it stops and we settle for agreed upon arbitrary ends and beginnings when really it's...always ongoing. We just step into the procession and think this is all when really it is. But this all is not restricted to us but inclusive of before, during, and after so there is only proximity relative to us or some other arbitrary spot segregated from the all. So as you broaden your awareness to include what was before before and after after you may find that the present is an even more rich and fertile place from which to grow in the ways you know you want and can. And maybe this just seems like so many words and while it is, it is more than this. It lets you in on a not so secret secret that makes the present just an ongoing sliding spot of time along an even larger line that maybe even makes a circle. But you can't repeat this unless you just want to go over the same old ground in the same old way and then only if this really is what will create what you want as you will know sometimes it does, but when you want a new result you choose new ground or new tools and or new seeds to plant and cultivate, depending on what... You know.

Intangibles: Accessing the Roots of Choice

The hypnotic language pattern below aims to access early stages of the decision-making process. In accessing these early stages, a client may enhance the decision-making process in three ways. First, they can better understand the ingredients that precede decisions. Second, they can recruit more useful resources that will enhance the effectiveness of decisions, developing deeper insight. Third, they can increase foresight, which better matches choice of resources to desired outcomes as a result of greater clarity about self, options, and goals.

Yes, trusting one's unconscious mind can be a very powerful aid in guiding one's life provided this guidance comes from the deepest source of knowledge within the self. I encourage utilizing our wisest, deepest, most knowing self. Sometimes, we find our life directed by unconsciously stored lessons or beliefs that are super-imposed on the deeper unconscious mind, leading to less informed or less effective decisions. Greater conscious awareness of unconscious processes can increase effective life direction, overriding influential but limiting beliefs that may be stored in the unconscious mind. By removing or nullifying effects of limiting beliefs stored in the unconscious, we can increase our ability to draw more fully from the wise self residing deep within the unconscious mind.

Everything that you see originated from what you did not see, see? And when you notice what you notice, realize…this is the end product, the result of things and events that began way before you notice the end result. You could trace back from the surface, going down deep below, or you could trace back before the surface, going way back to before you even noticed or felt anything about what you used to feel now. For example, this year's grass is more the result of last year's moisture than anything else. Yet you may not have thought about or noticed the profound effect this moisture was going to have when it was happening.

You could even trace the end result you see, the green grass, from the very tip down through the soil, finding and identifying all the ingredients that went into making this lovely grass grow. If you had a small camera and could burrow down below the surface, starting with the very top tip of the green grass, a single blade, tracing it down to where it enters the soil. You could then go below the ground to see the light brown stalk that goes even deeper still to become what is the root, these fine strands of tan that spread out to gain more and better access to the necessary ingredients allowing growth.

As you look around down there you can see the moisture that resides there and even the process of the roots taking it in. Further and perhaps deeper you can find the other nutrients, the needed ingredients that reside within the soil that the roots desire and take in, knowing it will allow the best growth. You could even see, if you used time-lapse images, this moisture and the nutrients with the soil being absorbed into the roots, being distributed through the entire blade of grass, combining with the sunshine from above to set in motion this most amazing process of remarkable growth. Noticing how the grass knows, knows and uses just the particular ingredients that it needs in just the right combinations that allow optimum growth and health. And it's interesting to know that at some level the grass knew, even before it grew this year that it was going to be a very good year since it already knew that it knew…and it has just what it needs to ensure this and did…identify and acquire the ingredients that certainly lead to the desired growth…desiring, planning, acquiring, growing…feeling this…gooood.

Flowing: Releasing the Past

The purpose of this pattern is to help release the listener-reader from ruminating about the past. While this hypnotic pattern involves time, the aim is to affect behavior; thus the pattern is included in this chapter about behavior. We often review the past and get mired in it, trying to gain something from it for our present use. Ideally, we use the past to derive beneficial principles and lessons for our present and future. The following language emphasizes letting go of the past after extracting beneficial content so that we can move on into the present and future more effectively.

The format used is a little different, being hypnotic language poetry (using the term loosely), followed by a more traditional hypnotic language script. While the concepts are what matters, a rhyme scheme exists within the poem. The rhyme scheme stops, however, at the point when the suggestion is presented to break free of the past and move toward the future. Absence of rhyme after several rhyming stanzas is intended to suggest breaking free of old patterns that loop and repeat rhyming schemes in one's own life.

> For those who hold on to the past
> Thinking it has something that will last
> It does, memories under glass
>
> Looking through the lens, convex.
> Waiting but just perplexed
> It remains still, dormant, decorative at best
>
> Perhaps belonging in a museum or in a tower
> That holds your past days or hours
> Something we all share but it does not flower
>
> Mourning the loss while it continues
> Climb the tower, glimpse a scape that moves
> Especially toward your future, views.
>
> What you rise above, relegated to a bin
> A has-been not a fluid now flowing
> Feel the pull of the current showing

There's a reason the waters flow
What awaits that's bigger, they know
The merging brings power from long ago

From deep within bubbling up,
Oozing, cascading breaking free
It's before before, aboriginally

Timeless yet now and then
All at once and one at a time
Be pulled, pushed, move on this

No impedance, only moving
Relentless knowing that it's going
Following to the future, always

And it is so interesting how there is…this natural system occurring in nature that arranges the small moving toward the big and the big toward the bigger. If you have ever looked at a map of the land in your state or your country or that of another country, you can be aware that by the time the map is made it already needs updating. Yet on this map there remains a constant: the flowing waters. Many features of the land represented by the map change but the waters maintain their ever-present system. These waters have a universal agreement that the smallest creeks will flow to a larger stream, which flows to a river, which perhaps then finds an even bigger river, wider, deeper and therefore more powerful and this then flows to an even bigger, more powerful, wider and deeper river that then flows to some grand body of water where a merging occurs making more now than was then so…bigger, better, more powerful and yet content to trust and simply rely on this system to feed and maintain this vast reservoir, distributed in ways from this.

And from a distance this reservoir may seem dormant or stagnant but it is never. There is ebb and flow in all parts from the point of entry to the outer edges where the shape takes form yet is, always in motion, dynamic. And when you think about yourself, you can find and feel your tributaries and to what do you pay tribute? From where do you flow and what flows to you and, more importantly, where are you flowing to?…And checking now to feel, well out into your future you can notice if there are any obstacles that need to be removed, allowing a smoother, easier flow for you to merge with and feel the immense immersion into the power within you, moving you in just the ways that you know you need, seeing and hearing, feeling this movement, this flow...through...the present to the future too...do and it's a big to do, isn't it now? And with each new...this much more powerful and determined to reach...and beyond.

Chapter 8
Hypnotic Language Script Addressing Smoking Cessation

This final section of hypnotic language presents a method of utilizing hypnosis for smoking cessation. This method has resulted from my work with clients who wanted to stop smoking. As I worked with these clients, each exhibited certain emotional and behavioral patterns involved in developing a smoking habit. I made use of these behavioral-emotional patterns in such a way as to help the client stop smoking. I will describe these patterns and their dynamics; then present a case using hypnosis to help the client stop smoking.

I think that in any addiction the addict is also addicted to an underlying emotional state associated with the item of addiction. For example, the gambling addict is addicted to the risk-taking they experience while gambling. The alcoholic is addicted to the state experienced while drinking alcohol. And the substance abuser or drug addict eventually develops a physical addiction such that absence of the substance craved leads to withdrawal symptoms. In the initial stages of addiction, I believe the individual develops this addiction to an emotional state associated with particular items used to bring about an altered state—whether slot machines, alcohol, drugs, or tobacco.

In the specific case of nicotine addiction, it seems the individual uses tobacco for one of two general reasons. The first reason is to change an unpleasant emotional state for the better. The second reason seems to involve enhancing or celebrating an already desirable state. The state from which an addict seeks release may be anxiety, boredom, or depression, for example. The individual smokes tobacco as a means of shifting out of such a state to experience a better state of relief or calm. While we know that nicotine is a physical stimulant, people often use it to relax mentally.

To illustrate enhancing a desirable state through smoking, when someone accomplishes an important goal, they may smoke a celebratory cigarette. When socializing with friends or family, for example, they may smoke a cigarette supposedly to enhance the already pleasant experience. Of the two motivators involved in smoking, the desire to shift from an unwanted to a more appealing state appears to be the stronger. I usually work first with negative emotions that trigger smoking as they seem to provide more leverage for behavioral change.

Identifying the two general motivators for smoking helps uncover a more specific sequence of variables that play out in nicotine addiction. The general dynamic involved in smoking hinges on situations smokers experience as either unpleasant or quite pleasant. The second stage involves the specific state experienced in reaction to this initial situation, which may range from anxiety to a sense of achievement or satisfaction, for example. The third step is lighting a cigarette with the ultimate goal, or fourth step, of shifting from or enhancing a particular state. Thus, the four steps that appear to be involved in maintaining a smoking habit are:

1. Experiencing a situation deemed unpleasant or especially pleasant;
2. Experiencing a reactive state associated with this initial situation;
3. Smoking itself;
4. Experiencing an altered desired state.

In the form of a flow chart, the sequence of events involved in sustaining smoking looks like this:

Event > State > Smoking > Desirable State

Those of you who are familiar with cognitive psychology may wonder where the cognitions enter into this smoking process. Cognitive psychology identifies one's thinking process as crucial in meaning making and as therefore contributing significantly to emotional states, beliefs, and behavior. I agree that the meaning-making process strongly influences emotional states, beliefs, and behavior. There seem to be two primary routes to personal change—one's thinking processes and one's emotional states. In smoking, the emotional states seem to be the driving force; thus, working with this dominant factor can make a significant difference in stopping the smoking habit.

Revisiting the smoking flow chart sequence, the intervention designed to stop smoking operates to change the sequence so that the individual experiences a more desirable emotional state on their own *before* smoking. Experiencing a more desirable emotional state prior to smoking then renders use of tobacco unnecessary because the desired outcome, formerly gained through smoking, is experienced without it. The new flow chart then looks like this:

Event > Desired Emotional State > Post-hypnotic Suggestions

A desired emotional state is accessed through the process of Meta-stating™ (Hall, 1995). Meta-stating™ is a process developed by Michael Hall. The therapist assists the client to raise their consciousness through a series of questions. Each successive level of consciousness allows more resourceful and constructive life management by the client. When used in therapy to stop smoking the result is that former smokers learn to alter their emotional state by themselves prior to smoking. The result is that they achieve a higher or better emotional state than tobacco ever provided. This change of state before smoking renders nicotine more than irrelevant: it makes it undesirable.

The individual learns that they had been pursuing a higher meta-state through smoking but that nicotine is actually a substance that dilutes or reduces experience of the desired meta-state. Tobacco becomes a substance that then threatens the desired higher state of consciousness rather than supposedly bringing about the desired state. Once the meta-state is established, as the response to an unpleasant or pleasant event, post-hypnotic suggestions—or *future pacing* as NLP refers to it—help the individual apply a new response style to each situation that formerly triggered smoking. Now that they can experience a better state than tobacco provided, they have more of what is desired. They can then more easily choose and maintain this new response style as its benefits far out-weigh harmful effects of nicotine. One last general statement about smoking and states of mind: I also believe that, in essence, higher states of consciousness preclude self-destructive acts such as smoking tobacco.

The following is a list of steps I use in smoking cessation intervention. I will elaborate on these in the case given below.

1. Establish the ultimate reason or purpose leading a client to want to stop smoking. This is usually a matter of loving self and/or others.
2. Identify all the situations in which this person smokes (while driving, working under a deadline, etc.).
3. Identify each emotional state that precipitates smoking (boredom, worry or anxiety, etc.).
4. Determine by questioning the client which of these identified emotional states is most likely to trigger smoking (worry, for example).
5. Raise the consciousness of the limiting emotional state through Meta-stating. Utilize post-hypnotic suggestions to make a new resourceful state the new response to an old situation that used to lead to smoking.
6. Utilize a new resource state as a replacement state for each of the old conditions that led to smoking.
7. Verify that the new resource state is more desirable for the client than the former act and emotional state created by smoking.
8. Utilize post-hypnotic suggestions from the near to the distant future to create a red carpet of success going forward.

Before presenting an example of this smoking cessation method, it is important to address the bigger picture. While people seem to smoke as a means of affecting their emotional states, at root these emotional states may originate in sources way beyond current life situations. It is vital that the therapist thoroughly assess the client's mental-emotional-physical history to determine if past factors involving parental or other relationships contribute to unwanted emotional states that trigger smoking.

Determine if the client is currently experiencing an ongoing, not situational, depression, anxiety, or some other pervasive unpleasant emotional state. If the roots of unwanted emotional states are ignored by the therapist, this intervention for smoking cessation is unlikely to be effective. A therapist increases a client's probability of success by identifying any extraneous variables involved that contribute to or help maintain smoking. If you identify some other unresolved emotional issues that contribute to the smoking habit, then you need to first help the client resolve these to reduce the issue down to just smoking. The finer the focus, the easier it becomes to produce success.

Prior to actually making an appointment with a client who wants to stop smoking, I also try to determine if this person is committed to stopping smoking. I make sure the client knows that if they have mixed feelings about not smoking, if any part of them likes to smoke and wants to keep smoking, or if they are trying to quit at someone else's insistence, the smoking cessation process will likely not be effective. Once we establish that this individual wants to stop smoking but has just not been able to achieve this, we make an appointment.

The example of smoking cessation that I am presenting involves a woman I'll name Gwen. Gwen came to me wanting to stop smoking after smoking one pack per day for nearly twenty years. She is in her late thirties and began smoking with friends during adolescence. I always ask the client the reason they started smoking, how long the habit has lasted, if they have ever quit, how they did so, for how long, and what caused them to resume smoking.

Gwen stated that she started to smoke so she could fit in with her peers and had never stopped smoking since. In the early stage of the intervention process, I also like to establish points that give the smoker a slightly different perspective, as a means of loosening the grip of nicotine. I mention that smokers very often start smoking in order to feel a sense of independence from their parents. It is ironic that the chosen method of experiencing independence actually results in dependence and self-harm.

I also mention research that indicates that, for each cigarette smoked, the smoker shortens life by about seven minutes, (although I've also heard five minutes and ten minutes.) Losing seven minutes of life per cigarette translates into 140 minutes per pack of cigarettes, or 2 hours and 20 minutes of life lost per pack. I expand upon this so the smoker cannot just think of smoking as indulging in a single cigarette. A one pack per day habit translates into nearly 16 hours of life lost per week, about 64 hours of life lost per month, and a life shortened by about 768 hours per year, which means you lose about 30 days or a whole month of your life per year when smoking one pack per day. In a decade you lose nearly 300 days and in two decades 600 days or 20 months—almost two years. I repeat these statistics slowly and wait for each round to take effect, observing the client's response. Sometimes I ask, "Did you know that?" after each round of numbers. Loss of life translates into leverage to help interfere with smoking, as smokers almost always state they want to quit in order to experience more time with loved ones or more time in various activities that hold importance for them.

The next step in this process is to determine the client's ultimate reason or purpose to stop smoking. This purpose will serve as leverage for the client to make the change from being a smoker to having more of what they really want. Usually, the most compelling reason someone finds to stop smoking is quality and length of life with loved ones. Determining the ultimate reason to stop smoking involves beginning with the client's stated reason for wanting to stop. You then ask the client, "As a result of having better health (for example), what will you then be able to experience that is even more important?" Maybe the client responds, "I'll be able to keep up with my wife and grandkids better." The therapist then follows up on this answer by asking, "And what makes this important to you?" or "What will you be able to experience as a result of that?"

This questioning process is somewhat like Meta-stating™ and somewhat like Core Transformation™ (Andreas & Andreas, 1994) questioning sequences. In this case, however, we are seeking to "meta-value" this person, identifying the highest value driving the desire to stop smoking. As the therapist, you continue asking the client what they will be able to experience that is even more important than the cited benefit of stopping smoking. "Meta-valuing" the client also brings needed emotional energy to the process as the client accesses emotions associated with the most valued aspects of life. This emotional energy can fuel the desired change.

I further verify with the client that, in order to smoke, they must disengage each time from contact with those they hold dear. The client always realizes this: they must disconnect from those they value most in order to engage in smoking, for each individual drag on a cigarette. This then adds up to a double loss through smoking, shortening life by a month a year *and* disconnecting from loved ones or valued activities for over two hours a day—lose now *and* lose later!

Now back to the specific case of Gwen. Once the preliminary history and general questions are answered by the client, we move to identifying the strongest purpose for stopping smoking. For Gwen, having more time with loved ones—husband, children, and soon-to-be-born grandchild—was her most compelling reason to give up cigarettes.

Once the ultimate purpose of stopping smoking has been identified, we then address situations in which Gwen smokes. Gwen says that she smokes in various situations at home and at work. She cites stress as a major trigger. She also cites smoking in response to boredom but also at times when she experiences a sense of accomplishment. Notice the two categories of avoiding a negative and enhancing a positive emotional state. These general categories of smoking triggers need to be dissected in order to understand their ingredients. Stress is such a general term it is hard to identify the necessary details about it that could promote change. I asked Gwen what she meant by stress and what emotions she experienced during stress. She identified anxiety, tension, and worry as the three factors that amounted to stress for her. The next step was identifying the most powerful of these ingredients. Gwen cited anxiety as the most powerful trigger for craving a cigarette.

Let's now turn to the boredom that moves Gwen to smoke. I have found over years of working with clients that boredom appears to be a distant or close cousin to depression. In the state of boredom there exists a sort of vacuum or absence of mental-emotional substance. Thus, boredom is a response or reaction to an absence, not necessarily a loss, but at least the absence of a state that had been most recently experienced This most recently experienced state may have been associated with some task. According to each client I've worked with, they report a mild sense of sadness accompanying boredom at its core.

This bored state seems to translate into a longing for something satisfying to place in the vacuum. It seems an unmet need exists when a person experiences boredom. It is an empowering experience when someone learns how to emerge from boredom into a desirable emotional state. The new desirable state seems to provide emotional comfort and may also offer a sort of behavioral traction allowing the individual to take constructive action toward a chosen goal.

Now we'll examine the desire to smoke in celebrating a sense of accomplishment. Almost immediately after accomplishing a meaningful goal, Gwen would want to smoke what amounted to a celebratory cigarette. I liked to point out to this client how interesting it is that, when some event goes well, she celebrates by smoking a life-shortening cigarette so that she would experience fewer such cherished moments. The act of smoking would make for fewer opportunities to feel the desired sense of accomplishment, since it cuts life short. (This last sentence purposely uses a vague term "it" cuts life short. Does "it" refer to smoking or to a sense of accomplishment? Though rather obvious, letting the client determine the meaning behind such ambiguity can add to the client's sense of empowerment as she makes the decision, taking more control over her life.) You can then ask the client, "So just what is it that you want more to accomplish more of?" This intervention of pointing out actions and consequences invites foresight and choice into a process that had been unthinking and habitual, thus loosening the chain of events involved in smoking.

After identifying and examining each of the circumstances and states that lead Gwen to smoke, we now narrow our focus to the one that exerts the most influence on smoking. She identified anxiety as possessing the most power to make her light up. Up to this point I have been inviting the client to move in and out of light trances through presented words and concepts; now we move into deeper trance work. This intervention follows the general process of Meta-stating™. I explain the general process and principles we will use to induce smoking cessation. I ask if she has any questions or concerns about hypnosis in general and our process in particular. Once any questions or concerns are addressed, we proceed to the actual intervention.

The following transcript is from my intervention sessions with Gwen. Taken as a guide, you can modify it to suit your client's situation and your own style. I begin by saying,

JB: The first step in changing your thinking, emotions, and choices is by starting with the old way you want to leave behind. To do this, let your mind drift back to find an example of when you felt anxiety and this led you to smoke. Just drift back through time and open the file you call "anxiety". And you may first find a good example of anxiety that led you to smoke then and then you may find another that is even more powerful. Just observe, notice, and let me know when you find and feel an example that truly represents you experiencing anxiety. You can just nod your head to let me know.

Gwen: [*She nods that she has found a strong example of anxiety that led her to smoke.*]

JB: Now that you have identified an example of anxiety, please allow yourself to step into the experience of anxiety so that you actually re-experience the anxiety. This will allow you to better release it. Go ahead and begin feeling the anxiety, mentally, emotionally, and physically. Step into the anxiety fully and notice how and where you feel it. Go right to the very center of the anxiety and immerse yourself in it and notice where you feel this. And where do you feel this physically Gwen?

Gwen: I feel the anxiety in my chest.

JB: How do you describe this sensation of anxiety you feel in your chest?

For clients who seem to have trouble finding descriptions of their physical sensations I usually offer a few examples of adjectives such as "tight" or "heavy," "loose" or "warm" that can be used to describe physical sensations. Gwen states that she feels a tightness and heaviness in her chest. I then ask her to feel and experience this anxiety fully, emotionally and physically. After several seconds, roughly five to ten, based on her body language, I say,

JB: Now imagine that every bit of this anxiety, the emotion and the physical sensation is totally and fully extracted from you. What do you now experience in the total absence of all anxiety?"

Gwen: [*Pauses briefly.*] I feel relief.

JB: Where do you feel this relief in your body?

Gwen: In my chest.

JB: Can you think of a word to describe the feeling in your chest?

Gwen: I notice a lightness in my chest.

I ask her to elaborate so she can more fully experience this new emotional-physical state. I ask her to describe this relief she experiences.

Gwen: My chest feels lighter and not so tight.

JB: [*To expand and deepen this new state.*] Allow this lightness to spread throughout your physical self from your scalp to your finger tips to your toes and all points in between, deepening this much more so that you feel this totally and completely through your entire self. And as you feel this relief and the lightness it brings to the absolute utmost, to the absolute maximum, what do you get to experience and what do you call this?

Gwen: Calm.

JB: Where do you feel this calm in your physical self, and how does this feel?

Gwen states she notices this calm feeling throughout her whole body and the feeling is "warm and light". I continue to invite her to spiral upwards to new and higher, stronger states along this path.

JB: When you feel this calmness as you do through your whole physical self and within your mind and whole being and you turn this up to the absolute maximum and step into this fully, going to the very center of this feeling and then to the very center of the very center where it is the strongest, cleanest, and most concentrated, what do you get to experience and what do you call this?

Gwen: Peace.

We continue this same progression of stepping into each state fully and totally, going to the very center of the very center, experiencing this state to the absolute utmost and then naming the state. Gwen reaches a state she calls "euphoria". This seems to be her ultimate meta-state, for it took her a moment to find a word to describe her experience. Knowing that there exists a place in our inner world that is experience beyond words, I always try to squeeze out one more meta-state.

I ask Gwen to fully and totally experience euphoria and when she experiences this to the absolute utmost.

> **JB:** What does this then allow you to experience and what do you call it?
>
> **Gwen:** [*Her facial expression shifts slightly and she seems puzzled.*]
>
> **JB:** Do you have a state of mind and emotion that you are experiencing but no word really describes it?
>
> **Gwen:** [*She nods in agreement.*]
>
> **JB:** [*I affirm.*] There are states of mind and awareness that exist that are sooo wonderful that we can't find words to describe them. It is just a great awareness of a wonderful experience that no words can truly describe. Just continue enjoying this experience and notice, is there any visual symbol that comes to mind that represents this feeling for you? It can be a person, place, thing, or color. Just let it come to you from within this feeling that is…beyond euphoria.

I always ask if the client can identify a visual symbol for whatever may be the highest meta-state achieved. If the client does not have a visual symbol, that is fine. But if she does, it can provide you with an additional tool for post-hypnotic suggestions to assist in stopping smoking. Gwen identified the color blue as her visual symbol for her ultimate meta-state. I asked her what shade, and she replied it was a light blue.

Now that Gwen had reached her ultimate meta-state and found a visual symbol or icon for it, it was time to apply this new resource to her old issue. First I wanted to establish this new state as far more important than smoking cigarettes and than any remotely positive state associated with smoking.

> **JB:** As you fully feel this beyond-euphoria feeling, don't you find that this is actually the very state that you had hoped to experience from smoking?
>
> **Gwen:** [*She nods in agreement.*]

JB: And don't you find that as you feel this beyond-euphoria feeling that if you were to smoke, that you would actually take away from this best feeling, diluting it and contaminating it?

Gwen: [*She again nods in agreement.*]

With the euphoric state established as the preferred one and Gwen well associated into the state, we then moved to reconfigure past events when smoking had occurred.

JB: [*Inviting her to remain within the ultimate meta-state.*] Now think back to the original situation in which you had been feeling anxiety, except now, continue feeling and experiencing this wonderful state, beyond euphoria with the light blue color you see. Notice as the situation happens and you continue feeling this great feeling, what do you find yourself choosing to do instead of what you used to do?

Gwen states that she sees herself just keeping relaxed and decides to just handle the situation and go on about her business without smoking.

JB: How does this feel as you see yourself doing this?

Gwen: Wonderful!

I then elaborate a bit and invite Gwen to consider more details about the new state applied to the old situation.

JB: Notice how this feels to continue feeling relaxed and wonderful. And notice how this just naturally leads to choices that let you feel more....Notice the opportunities and possibilities to use this feeling and how it only leads to more of it. Notice how you find you deal with others differently from this feeling and way of being...and how you feel inside and how you feel about yourself. How *does* this feel?

I like to get feedback and invite a client to add details and additional dimensions to their state, to sense its applications and consequences for more enriched experience. I find such enriched experience gives more foundation, stability, and endurance to the new resource state as this becomes more intricately connected with the client's internal and external environment. Gwen stated that she felt "very good" as she observed her new state's influence on old situations.

We then looked into the future, applying it to various anticipated circumstances.

JB: While continuing to feel this wonderful, beyond-euphoria feeling and this appealing light blue, see yourself in your future, with this feeling in a situation that would have in the past resulted in you feeling anxious and smoking, but now...you feel this beyond-euphoria feeling instead. What do you see yourself feeling and doing differently?

Gwen: I see myself feeling very good, very relaxed, and just handling the situation, confident, and just moving on.

I ask how this feels to her and she says it feels "great". I then asked Gwen to identify two more specific situations in which she would have felt anxiety and would have smoked. She looked at these old situations through her new resource state, beyond euphoria. We then identified responses that came to mind as a result of this new state and explored how she felt about her new feelings and options.

Each reconfiguring of old situations and emotional-behavioral responses went well, so we then moved on to the next step. This involves general, blanket applications of the new state and behavior to the future. The more an individual can associate a new state and behavioral repertoire to various conditions of the internal and external environment, the more likely this new state of being will take root. You might say we are building new neurological pathways that will be activated and utilized in the future in response to situations that formerly triggered anxiety and smoking.

I invite Gwen to expand her awareness of the new state beyond-euphoria with its associated blue color, and apply this to her future.

JB: While experiencing this feeling of beyond-euphoria, allow yourself to look well into your future, days, weeks, months, and years. All the while experiencing this feeling and the light blue, see yourself in your future present free of cigarettes and how good this feels. Notice how this feeling and the light blue extend well out into your future and even beyond so that you see and feel this feeling all around and within you as far out into your future as you can see and beyond so that you are and will have been experiencing this feeling and you are and have been free of cigarettes and how this feels…now. And how does this feel?

Gwen: Fantastic!

I like to make one final checking statement to a client that aims to make smoking and this new ultimate meta-state mutually exclusive, binding the new meta-state as the preferred choice in response to what had been anxiety-provoking situations. We had already established that smoking shortens life, that this meta-state is the desired state, and that smoking would, in the client's estimation, dilute and contaminate the meta-state.

JB: As you feel this best of all feelings, this beyond-euphoria feeling and all that it brings to you, is there any situation in which you would exchange this best feeling for a contaminating, life-shortening cigarette?

Gwen: [*She pauses for a moment while she thinks.*] NO! [*Emphatically*]

JB: How does this feel?

Gwen: Great!

Once we finished this process and Gwen came out of trance, we discussed her experience. I invited her to make any comments or ask questions. Gwen had no questions or comments; she was clearly enjoying the pleasant altered state she had achieved. I invited Gwen to savor this new experience and the well-being it brings. Over 18 months later, Gwen is still free of cigarettes and has made other healthy lifestyle adjustments such as regular exercise and eating healthier foods. She reported no significant withdrawal symptoms.

We now reach the conclusion of this material on advanced hypnotic language. Several stages were presented to provide an understanding of the concepts and applications of hypnotic language. In the initial phase, cognitive, perceptual, and human development concepts were presented and arranged into an interacting hierarchy. This hierarchy provides an understanding of how we make meaning in life and live out this meaning. More centrally to this book's material, this hierarchy provides opportunities for the therapist to intervene with hypnotic language in helping clients make personal change.

Once we established the variables and dynamics of the foundation of meaning-making, we explored various ways to assess the client's level of awareness and functioning. This then provides a template through which to view the client and to tailor hypnotic language patterns to their cognitive-perceptual-developmental structure. Many case illustrations and free-standing language patterns were provided as examples, along with the reasoning preceding the chosen intervention. Hopefully, this glimpse into the structure and application of hypnotic language provides you with a better understanding and ability to utilize this unique and potent form of psychotherapy.

Appendix
The Milton Model:
Hypnotic Language Patterns

At the beginning of this book, I made reference to Dr Milton H. Erickson. He developed and utilized a unique manner of providing psychotherapy for his clients through the use of hypnosis. In particular, he utilized hypnotic language to great effectiveness. Extensive study of Erickson's skills and applications of hypnotic language led to the development of the *NLP Milton Model*. The Model allows other therapists to identify hypnotic language categories and utilize them in their own unique ways.

The collection of identified hypnotic language categories, known as the Milton Model, is presented within this Appendix. While there may exist a few additional, more sophisticated categories of the Milton Model, the collection that follows covers the vast majority.

The principle that runs through these hypnotic language categories is that each contains a form of language that is purposefully vague. This vagueness provides a sort of blank canvas for the listener to fill in their own personal meanings. To fill in the blanks, the listener goes into a trance while searching within for the "filler" materials. Each of the Milton Model categories listed below is described in terms of its grammatical structure followed by several examples illustrating the style of the category. The overall Model provides a way of inducing trance, deepening trance, or assisting clients in discovering and applying solutions to their problems.

Mind Reading

A statement claiming that you know the thoughts or feelings of another person without identifying how you know. These kinds of statements help induce an internal focus and resulting trance.

- "I know what you're thinking."
- "As you sit here, I can tell you hear I feel..."
- "Since you're feeling doubt, go ahead and use that doubt to take a closer look at the situation, as I know you're curious, to find more detailed and useful information."
- "I know you understand these so you can make your own now."

Lost Performative

A general value statement about self, life, or others, that contains no source for the value statement. A statement that suggests wrong or right, good or bad, but the source or reference for this statement is lost. Utilizing lost performatives provides a general outline or guide for the client to follow toward a resource and utilize it.

- "I know what you're thinking and it's a good thing to think."
- "Conflict is terrible."
- "I'm a bad person."
- "It's good to feel curious."

Cause and Effect

A statement implying that one action, event, thing, or person causes a particular outcome. This sort of language makes for a good reframe opportunity. Cause-and-effect patterns can also work well for linguistic time-lining or future pacing. Cause-and-effect patterns often contain the words "if", "then", "makes", or "because". Using such patterns you can link choices in the present to desired outcomes in the future. At some fundamental level of a "problem", the client uses a cause-and-effect reversal, a sort of dyslexic logic. Addressing this by reversing the reversal, clients can remove themselves from the "problem" and move toward a solution.

- "I know what you're thinking and it's a good thing to think because then you will know more of what you want to know more of."

- "You used to think that choosing to eat that piece of cake meant you were free, but it really limited and enslaved you, making you the way you do not want to be. And now *not* eating that piece of cake means you are free to choose anything you want, feeling and doing what you really want to do more, feeling and being the way you really want to be and are now, free and in control as you choose."
- "It's important that you continue not expressing your true thoughts and feelings to the people in your life so that you will never really know who your true friends are."
- "He did not go on a drinking binge because she divorced him; she divorced him because he's the kind of person who chooses to go on drinking binges."
- "You may think that you caused your mother's behavior and that you could then prevent it if you behaved just right. But the truth is that your mother's behavior motivated *your* behavior because, after all, which came first? It's just that after a long time of your mother starting things and you reacting, you forgot where it all started because it went back and forth, back and forth, but never forth and back. You know, sometimes people accidentally exchange the first letters of two words and get it wackbards, K.O.? But it's not accurate, only separately and not together. But then you could get back and words, leaving some words back in your past to more forward into your future with new meaning that you really already knew, didn't you?"

Complex Equivalence

A statement identifying two separate things and suggesting they are equal in some way or ways. Complex equivalence patterns offer an explanation of events and another opportunity for re-framing and future pacing. For example, in response to the client who states, "Everything is my fault," the therapist might respond, "Well, doesn't that give you an immense amount of power? I can see how your incredible might might concern you. I guess believing that everything's your fault is really your error, or you just want to learn how to better use this immense power you possess."

- "I know what you are thinking and it's a good thing to think because then you will know more of what you want to know more of, which means you gain more control and can decide for yourself what it is you want."
- "I know you are wondering how you made this change that you wanted and it concerns you that you don't know. But this means that your unconscious mind has already integrated new ways into your new routine and you can relax and trust your unconscious mind will continue this."
- "It's O.K. that you don't know how you made those changes that you feel good about because it means that your unconscious mind made those changes and your unconscious mind knows more than your conscious mind, so you really know more than you don't know."

Presuppositions

Statements using an unspoken assumption to then make a statement about the assumption. This spoken statement assumes something about past circumstances or future choices or outcomes. Presuppositions also leave out specifics. Presuppositions send the listener on a search to fill in the implied blanks. In some sense, a presupposition resides beneath all statements.

- "And you can use this to make even more of the changes you really want."
- "As your awareness increases, you can begin."
- "Only practice this as much as you want to improve."
- "Will you have stopped half-sabotaging yourself by then?"
- "And I know you'll decide on whatever is most needed because you always scratch where it itches the most."
- Combining with a double bind: "And which of these choices do you think feels best?"
- "This is one of the most important things you'll ever remember."

Universal Quantifiers

Statements utilizing words to make universal generalizations with no reference to the source. Universal quantifiers always make a general statement of fact. Words used in this category include "always", never", and any word that is a general catchall such as "they" or "it". The function serves to broaden the listener's awareness. Universal quantifiers resemble lost performatives but contain no reference to values.

- "It always helps…"
- "They say…"
- "Everybody's that way."
- "And now everything you notice from this point forward can be thought of in terms of this new state you know and feel and use and all the many opportunities and the many ways…"

Modal Operators

You can utilize words that suggest possibility or maybe you should utilize words that suggest necessity. When made by clients, modal operator statements often reveal past limiting beliefs or present resourceful beliefs. Modal operators set rules and frames for life. Some presupposition underlies each modal operator. An unspoken consequence for the preventative strategy of necessity operators suggests that something bad will happen if you do not do what you ought or should, have to or must do. Some positive consequence is implied when you do what you can or will, want to or get to do.

- "And you can begin to utilizing all the new learnings."
- "And you should, you know, remove such limits on yourself so that you can."
- "And when you decide you will, you will because you can, you know—just like you always knew you should but now want to for yourself."
- "You can think about the things you think you should have done in your past, and you can think about the things in your future you can do so you will have…the future you want because you don't want a future that you look back on full of *should haves*. Instead, you want a future full of *cans* because you will…this building energy into action."

Nominalizations

Isn't the word nominalization a nominalization? Well, we could go on forever about that loop. Nominalizing freezes a process word or a verb into a noun, often by taking away the "–ing." Nominalizing also labels behavior, thoughts, persons, or processes. Nominalizing reveals all-or-nothing thinking by using just a single word to describe a very complex process among an infinite number of other complex processes existing along a continuum. Hypnotic language utilizes nominalizations in two ways. First, hypnotic language de-nominalizes, thawing words, concepts, and thoughts to allow the return of active choice. Second, hypnotic language purposely nominalizes words to convey a general category to the listener. This then allows the listener to draw on and utilize this general category any way they choose.

- "Using new learnings creates new outcomes."
- "And you can begin piecing things together."
- "And you love loving, don't you?"
- "When expectations come into contact with all the things that are possible, which is everything, then there are no expectations, just all possibilities, and nothing is not everything, is it?"
- The statement, "I am depressed" becomes a question. "How are you depressing yourself?" or "How do you do depression?"

Unspecified Verbs

A verb may leave doubt about the process or experience described. Such verbs hang in the air, not clearly attached to any fully specified process or outcome. They presuppose readiness, grant permission, and send the listener on a search for how, when, and where to locate the action. These statements suggest action but by whom and applied to what may be unclear.

- "Seeing…feeling…knowing…using…creating."
- "And you can, of course."
- "Feeling good…"
- "Beginning now."
- "Knowing and using…knowing…"

- "You can discover."
- "Making changes."

An addendum: as clients consistently speak in hypnotic language themselves, be on the "listen-out" for unspecified verbs. If a client says, "I'm just dragging everywhere I go," this unspecified verb "dragging" may refer to some part of themselves in conflict. Ask them, "What are you dragging everywhere you go?" Elicit the inner dynamic of whatever they say they're dragging. Gain an understanding of the dragging part's thoughts, feelings, and needs. Treat the dragging part by first exploring its dynamics, then helping the client tend its needs.

Tag Questions

Questions added after a statement in order to decrease resistance and increase compliance, like "won't you?" Research suggests that it is a slightly more challenging mental task to negate than to affirm. In response to a negative tag question, you first have to affirm and then you negate after, don't you? You have to play the verbal recording in the positive form in your mind, then add the negating aspect. Tag questions also serve to tamp down an already agreed upon change. You can also use tag questions to do time-lining, haven't you?

- "And nothing's not everything, is it?"
- "And you won't do it until your unconscious is ready, now will you?"
- "And when you get there and you recognize what's happening, you will have done just as you please, won't you?"
- "You can stop that whenever you want, will you not?"
- "You can't not find somebody in the future, can you?"
- Try these sentences with various time-oriented tags, won't you?

Lack of Referential Index

This occurs when a statement leaves out something, leaving you to wanting to ask, "What?" Essentially the other half of the statement or the details are missing either as to the application or what the statement refers to. If a client says, "I'm dissatisfied," with what or whom and in what way are they dissatisfied? They make sentences like these using unspecified nouns and pronouns with no attached value. It makes me crazy!

- "I always want everything just so-so." You might say, "So-so what?" or, "You mean you just want everything mediocre?"
- "And you can use this to make even more of the changes you really want."
- "And you can…"
- "You just want to feel happy."
- "It's that feeling, you know."
- "It works well."

Another form of sentence without referential index occurs when the first half of a statement contains two subjects and the second half of the statement makes reference to one subject without specifying which.

- "So you think you're talking about your father and feeling guilty, but you're really not."
- "I realize that when you do this, that happens, but it does not have to."
- "You can decide to do this or you can decide to do that, which is better."
- "I noticed I drink more water when it's cold."
- "I sure hope I sleep well tonight and I'm sure you feel the same."
- "Walking with your wife and feeling good go hand in hand."

Comparative Deletions

A statement in which a comparison is made between two or more items but the reference is left out. The person, thing, process, or standard used to compare is not there. Very often these comparative deletions contain a word ending in "–er" which makes them better. Sometimes the comparison contains a superlative, which makes it best.

- "Now just imagine how you will use this in your future, as best you can."
- I know you are thinking, and it's a good thing to think and maybe even better to know what's best."
- "You can decide to do that or you can decide to do this, which is better."
- "It could be done more or less, but it's best that you decide."
- "That sure is better."

Pacing Current Experience

This is a statement describing the client's external experience by using undeniable facts. This process helps gain rapport and also invites the listener to go inside self, verifying these indisputable details you provide. To pace current experiences, just draw on observable aspects that you know the client is currently experiencing. You could think of pacing current experience as combining mind reading with future pacing, and then imagine what you can come up with!

- "As you read this material, sitting or standing, I know you are carefully moving your eyes across the page, seeing, thinking, and realizing much."
- "As you sit there on this couch, just allow yourself to get into a comfortable position as you know how to do this and have done so well before."
- "As you notice your feet flat on the floor, you may feel the material of your socks and you may notice your hips and back nicely supported by the chair while you breathe, noticing that the air you inhale feels cooler than the air you exhale. And then you may notice that you notice that your breathing just naturally slows, growing deeper and slower, collecting energy as you inhale and releasing tension as you exhale...collecting... releasing...collecting...releasing to become more and more relaxed with each breath you release."

Double Binds

These statements offer the illusion of choice, usually through the word "or". But each choice is in keeping with an overall desired outcome. You could think of the double bind as referring to the "how" to accomplish an already decided on "what". Double binds can address behavior, beliefs, states, and/or time, whatever you decide will bring the most beneficial change.

- "Now you could read this information on double binds and find that you become very accomplished, or you could just practice writing and saying them to develop mastery."
- "You can continue to feel sleepy and realize that this allows your unconscious mind to pay that much more attention to what I'm saying, or you can become that much more alert and pay full attention to what I'm saying."
- "You can call her and find out she hasn't changed, or you can let her call and then you'll know she really has changed."
- "Do you want him to do these things because he loves you or because he loves you?"
- "And you can keep all of your doubt and experience the diluting effect it has on reaching and experiencing your goal, or you can release all of your doubt to experience the maximum, which is better. And of course you don't have to keep the full benefits, do you?"
- "Sooner or later, or now and then."
- "You can do this some of the time and get some of the benefits, or you can do this more and get more of the benefits, whichever you want more of and however you choose to use your control."
- "And you may wonder which of your hands feels more relaxed, maybe your left or maybe your right or maybe it's just wherever you notice, you feel the most relaxed."
- "It's O.K. not to tell me everything about this experience. I trust you'll only tell me what you decide you want me to know is most important."
- "Only practice this as much as you want to get better."

Conversational Postulate

A question posed in such a way that it requires a yes or no answer. The answer, either yes or no, essentially requires the listener to move toward the desired outcome. The question leaves a sort of unspoken blank (the desired response) that resembles a presupposition.

- "When you feel how you want to feel, will it matter why you didn't?"
- "Is something considered new five years after it began?"
- "Is there ever just one drop of rain?"
- "It feels good to feel good, doesn't it?"
- "And you can, can you not?"
- "You know exactly how now, don't you?"

Extended Quotes

Statements in which it is not clear where one quote leaves off and another begins. Extended quotes from a variety of sources, where one leads into another, can effectively dissociate the listener. This can also provide an effective vehicle for an embedded suggestion. You can also link one quote after another, very slowly leading up to your point. Delaying the point you want to make can increase the mental receptivity or "structure hunger" of the listener. By presenting an extended quote, you provide the ground of the perception first; then you provide the figure.

- "This friend of mine was telling me about a coworker's husband who was going through a tough time and all the while she was telling me I was listening. And finally she said, 'I can see you hear I feel more and more uplifted and confident that the solution is at hand'."
- "My second cousin was telling me about my first cousin once removed a very hot container from the oven and suddenly remembered, just before, that she needed to return a phone call to her mother who then remembered she'd told her about her husband's recent trip out of town on business and how he'd learned from his boss to make sure to use oven mitts."
- "Your situation reminds me of another client whom I knew who told me how he wanted to figure out what to do that would work best. He asked many people and looked for as many ideas as he could find. He told me about this one day when he was visiting some friends out of town and they decided to order a pizza to be delivered. He told me that these friends told him about this pizza they had recently tried. It was a really new sort of pizza with a certain kind of crust and certain ingredients and

they suggested to him that he would like it, so they ordered it and when the delivery person got there he had the exact change ready."

- "Yesterday a client was telling me that he can't stand to sit and I thought no truer words were ever spoken. Of course he can't stand to sit. These are mutually exclusive. When you do one, you can't do the other. And getting stuck in between the two would really get tiresome on your legs and back. Just what do you get confused about doing that tries to do two things at once and ends up only tiring, and what would you prefer?"

Selectional Restriction Violation

A statement in which living qualities are attributed to inanimate objects; personification. This kind of statement appeals to the infantile level of thinking that was present at the time the problem was likely formulated. Selectional restriction violations can also sidestep resistance (fear) by dissociating the listener from the issue and inviting a more playful, resourceful exchange. In addition, you can often address the unconscious part that constitutes the problem with these kinds of statements.

- "As your anxiety lessons, what does it teach you?"
- "It's the alcohol talking."
- "Time marches on and change is afoot and with each step, as your foot touches the ground, grow more deeply relaxed as you move toward your ultimate solution."
- "As you think about the blackboards that were present in the classes you were in, in school, you can think about all the information that was written on them. The different subjects and different teachers as the same room was used to teach different subjects with the blackboard used to display so much information and so many answers from the chalk used to write. You can think about that blackboard and how much it has learned over time and knows and you can think about the blackboard inside of you and how much information has been displayed and how many answers...."
- The reference to any specific educational level is left off so that the listener can search for just the right place and time to find the

information. If you knew the approximate time period of the problem or the level of the solution you could reference this as well, which would be elementary, wouldn't it?

Ambiguity

In some sense this category represents the essence of hypnotic language, ambiguity. Hypnotic language in the Ericksonian tradition is purposely ambiguous so that the listener can fill in and apply the necessary specifics that only the listener knows. In the case of this specific category of ambiguity, two purposes are served. Ambiguity confuses and dissociates the client from the problem at hand me a sheet of paper. Didn't that jar you a bit? And we were talking about, oh yes, the other function of ambiguity that serves to frame a blank canvas for the listener to paint on as they choose. Notice how ambiguity can disconnect from the problem of the past and from this point forward to the solution. There are four types of ambiguity: phonological, scope, syntactic, and punctuation.

A. *Phonological*—In essence, puns:

- "Instead of no end in sight, now it's no end insight."
- "Bored with the stationary and the usual way, he used a pencil lead him to write a letter do whatever she needs."
- "At lunch I had a salad with lettuce decide together what to do."
- "The other day I was driving along the road and took a U-turn your life in whatever direction you know you need to go."
- "It's important to get a good view of the problem from a higher perspective so you can overlook it well, but be sure you don't want to overlook the solution."
- "When she felt the felt she felt…deeply…relaxed."
- "Those thoughts can grow faint and pass out…of your mind completely."
- "Some people go camping to relax and stay in tents."
- "Growing tired of the now confining routine, he decided to move to Newark."
- "I went a week strong, it was a strong week."
- "It's just a nominal fee, which is different than a phe-nominal."
- "By the way, they had to find a way to weigh the whey."

You can think of many more examples on your own but find the limit because inflicting too many of these on others can be punishing.

B. *Scope*—The ambiguous range and application of the words to each other within a sentence:

- "The other day I was in a store wearing a tee shirt and the label was irritating my neck. My wife offered to tear it off."
- "You might think you'll fail by taking on that new project, but you'd be wrong."
- "He is an agitator."
- "They are mowing shoes."
- I don't know how deeply you will decide to go into trance in order to find what you want, but you will."
- "Yesterday I drove my car with tennis shoes on."
- "He told me that his wife told him that he never listens to her, which of course is impossible."
- "This morning they made pancakes in their pajamas."
- "Some people dream of really achieving their goals and the feeling it will bring, but I wouldn't dream I'd do it."
- "Recently I was in a store that sells all kinds of things. From somewhere off in the distance a few aisles away, I guess, I could hear an infomercial playing on the TV and the spokesperson said, 'It only takes a few moments of your time in the microwave.' And I knew this was false advertising because there is no microwave big enough for me to get in, and if there was I wouldn't."

I had fun putting these together and you might as well.

C. *Syntactic*—The application of a particular word within the sentence is ambiguous. To construct this, add an "-ing" to a verb and follow it with a noun. The other way to make syntactic ambiguity is to nominalize a noun:

- Policing police
- Smoking turkeys
- Relaxing times
- Driving tires
- Roofing men

- Counting crows
- Collecting bugs

D. *Punctuation*—Punctuation ambiguity consists of run-on sentences, improper pauses, or fragments.

- "You must make sense, so you can...."
- "You can see and then notice the feeling that allows..."
- "Letting go..."
- "Once you've embraced you can..."
- "When you think about the ways you used to...instead now how you can...and the feeling that moves you."

Utilization

Utilizing events that happen while interacting with the listener. This includes incorporating sounds, smells, actions, sights, or sensations that occur naturally within the process. Usually these are unplanned, spontaneous events and responses.

- I was working with a client who tended to lose his temper with his fiancée. We discussed the details of how he lost his temper, when, and for what reasons. We then identified how he often assumed some information about his fiancée or filled in missing pieces of information while his fiancée communicated with him (notice the closure effect). It seems to work fairly well to identify certain crucial points in the development of anger and insert questions by the anger-prone person in place of the previous irritating assumptions. While I was explaining this to him, he looked a bit confused. Right then he said, "So when I'm feeling confused or don't know some specific bit of information, I should just listen carefully to the person and then..." Since he was in the process of demonstrating the point, I cut him off and said, "Exactly, that's exactly it!" He paused and went inside himself to process this, then began to smile in amazement. He spontaneously went over the process he just experienced several more times in sequence, each time with pleasant surprise. This was absorbed by his mind and he used it from that point forward.

- As another example, when you and a female client are just finishing up a session, and, as she searches through her purse for her keys, you ask: "It's interesting how we always find when we know what we're looking for, isn't it?"
- I very often find that during a session that someone outside the room, down the hallway, says something that can be worked into the session. Maybe we're trying to establish some healthy boundaries for the client in a relationship and suddenly down the hall someone yells, "No!" Then I say, "Now that's exactly it," or "She sure knows how, doesn't she?"
- You can incorporate what might seem like interruptions or disturbances of various kinds into the session. Just keep an open mind and search for ways to make an association between the stimulus and the client's goals at the moment or with the big picture. Consider what to do examples or what not to do examples.

Analogue Marking

This involves utilizing one or more of the five senses to emphasize a point while talking or listening. Doing this can help a listener take in the information more easily because you make it STAND *OUT*. Ways of doing analogue marking can include some repeated reference at a crucial point. You might use sounds, voice alterations, facial expressions, or tangible items. This marking can also take the form of shifts of posture, body part location, and/or movement such as raising your hand or touching some specific item. Repeating this, this, this several times can also make it more memorable. Analogue marking is like a spotlight illuminating a crucial point.

- Sometimes when the client is in the process of leaving behind old ways and adopting new ones, I will pick out some item to associate with separating the two. For example, when a client was changing eating habits, I alternately touched my pen to my little finger and my forefinger and said, "It will be important for you to remember what to leave out [*touched pen to little finger*] and what to include [*touched my pen to my forefinger*]. I repeated this about three times then and found several more opportunities to emphasize this point in the same way.

You may also look for and listen for certain actions the client displays associated with the new way of thinking, feeling, and behaving. Maybe a client clears her throat each time she starts describing her resource state. You can then ask a question, wanting her to invoke her resource state to answer you and clear your throat at the end of your question, cueing her to access the resource state. Analogue marking can go in both directions, from you to the client (touching pen to fingertip) or from the client to you and then back to the client (clearing your throat to cue the resource state).

Embedded Commands

Such statements directly suggest what to do, so you will embed them in a larger sentence. Milton Erickson often utilized embedded commands. As with each of these hypnotic language categories, be sure you establish rapport with the listener and decide the necessary depth of trance for this strategy to be effective. Also, you will want to alter your voice for presenting these embedded commands. Notice how an embedded command becomes effective through lowering and slowing your voice when speaking key words.

- "Of course you are not going to use any of these until *your unconscious* mind is ready now."
- "As you think about your feet…you can *notice* your toes…each of them on each of your feet. You can also *notice* the arches of your feet…the tops of your feet…and within your feet…there are many fine muscle fibers present. You can *notice* these as well and scan from toes *to heel*."

When you construct embedded command sentences you *allow yourself* more opportunities to find *solutions* directly.

- "You *may notice how* when you went shoe shopping in the past, *you might* look at the top of the shoe, the sole, and certainly the color to decide but most important, you *only keep what fits*."

Maybe you can construct an embedded command by starting with the command and forming a sentence around it from the beginning to the end and then use it.

- For example, start with the embedded command "You want to now." Then think of what you want to now put at the beginning of the sentence. Maybe you could say, "Given that you now *make your own choices*…you can change when *you want to now*." Often embedded commands follow words like "and", "when", "then", "so that". or "notice". Embedded commands may include the word "now" at the very end so they become more compelling.
- "Notice how you *do this now* and then notice how you *do then too*."

Spelling

In the process of delivering hypnotic language patterns, I've noticed that you can invite the listener on an internal search if you s-p-e-l-l a crucial word in your language pattern. Spelling key words invites the client to place more focus on this word, then they k-n-o-w what you mean. You can also use spelling effectively when you want to differentiate between homonyms such as the p-e-a-c-e that you feel.

Compound Suggestions

These phrases are what first appear to present as paradoxes. This arrangement invites the listener to focus on the phrase in order to decode the meaning. In the process of focusing on the phrase you can increase the application and experience of the words

- Still moving
- I can't stand to sit.
- A little big
- That's odd even
- "You can allow those thoughts to begin slowing faster, an ever faster slowing…."

Linking language

This form of hypnotic language combines pacing current experience or utilization linked to specific words, and you can as you read this. Three types of linking language exist—conjunctions, disjunctions, and adverbial clauses or implied causes.

Conjunctions, words such as "and", provide the link between resources or between resources and their application.

- "As you sit here reading this sentence, you can begin to wonder what applications exist and you can wonder about the benefits and begin imagining and experiencing."

Disjunctions combine several options under the umbrella of a single desired outcome. The outline of this pattern looks like X and X and X but Y. The diagram of this pattern looks like offering the client option A, B, or C, though each is an example of generally desired behavior X. Maybe you will find it easiest to relax with your feet flat on the floor or maybe you'll choose to keep your eyes open or maybe close your eyes and find that you decide to feel your hands relax first. It describes the many ways that you can either see, hear, feel, or simply do what you know but you can use this technique just fine anyway you like. You can think of this disjunction category as being a multiple bind rather than a double bind. It is somewhat like a suggestion covering all possibilities.

Adverbial clauses or *implied clauses* often link resources to an outcome in a time bind that implies cause.

- "Since you can now assert yourself as you need to, you can then manage this meeting effectively."
- "Once you find that most comfortable position that you know is just right, you can fully release all tension and just relax as you know how."
- "It turns out that your parents really just told you and sold you a bill of goods that was not good, it was totally inaccurate. But you did not know any better so believed it. And then all those decisions you made and the bad results you got were just based on the false information your parents gave you, so that really you are what they never told you, you know? And won't it be interesting finding out and using this rich collection?"

Bibliography

Andreas, C. & Andreas, T. (1994) *Core transformation: Reaching the wellspring within*. Real People Press: Moab, UT.

Burton, J. (2003) *States of equilibrium*. Carmarthen, Wales: Crown House.

Burton, J. & Bodenhamer, B. (2000) *Hypnotic language: Its structure and use*. Carmarthen, Wales: Crown House.

Festinger, L. (1957) *A theory of cognitive dissonance*. New York: Harper and Row.

Frankl, V. (1973) *Man's search for meaning*. New York: Simon & Schuster.

Hall, L.M. (1995) *Meta-states: A domain of logical levels, self-reflexive consciousness in human states of consciousness*. Grand Junction, CO: ET Publications.

Keagan, R. (1983) *The evolving self*. Cambridge, MA: Harvard University Press.

Piaget, J. (1965) *The child's conception of the world*. Patterson, NJ: Littlefield, Adams.

Rossi, E. (2002) *The psychobiology of gene expression*. New York: W.W. Norton.

Wertheimer, M. (1912) Experimentelle studien über das sehen von bewegung. *Zeitschrift für, Psychologie*, 60, 312–378.

Index

Keagan, R   3, 223

lack of referential index   209–210
linking language   220
lost performative   204, 207

meaning-making   3–5, 11, 94,
    201
metaphor   1–2, 75, 77, 78, 81, 83,
    85, 103, 110–112, 114, 117, 118,
    123, 128, 152, 161, 162, 165,
    167, 173, 177, 178, 179
meta-stating   189–194
Milton model   203–221
mind reading   203, 211
modal operators   207

nominalisations   208

pacing current experience   211,
    220
perceptual level   4, 10, 11, 18, 21,
    110
perceptual position   9, 10
pessimism   35, 58
Piget, J   3, 43–63, 223
presupposition(s)   23, 44, 206, 207,
    212
processing
    first tier   1, 2, 10 et seq
    second tier   3, 25
    third tier   3, 43
    fourth tier   59–61
proximity   25–30, 144, 181

reframing   1–2, 52, 146,
    204–205
relationship(s)   20, 31, 37, 40, 46,
    47, 50, 56, 91, 94, 105, 106, 134,
    149, 190, 218
resistance   35, 99–100, 170, 209,
    214
resource state   10, 17, 66, 83, 121,
    190, 198, 199, 219
Rossi, E   89, 94, 223

selectional restriction violation
    214
self-worthy   120, 149
similarity   32, 33, 97
smoking cessation   35, 187–201
spelling   220
stress   73–74, 193

tag questions   209
time distortion   142, 145
timeline   29, 34, 53, 57, 128
trance state   1, 32, 40, 50, 67, 142,
    145
transductive logic   27, 56–58
trauma   27, 32, 43, 75–76, 78

unspecified verbs   208–209
utilization   158, 127, 220
values   5, 49, 71, 86, 87, 91,
    207
weight loss   74, 151–154,
    179–180
Wertheimer, M   25, 223